SEVEN sensible STRATEGIES for drug-free kids

J. Stuart Rahrer

Child & Family Press
Washington D.C.

CWLA Press is an imprint of the Child Welfare League of America. The Child Welfare League of America (CWLA), the nation's oldest and largest membership-based child welfare organization, is committed to engaging all Americans in promoting the well-being of children and protecting every child from harm.

CHILD WELFARE LEAGUE OF AMERICA, INC.
440 First Street, NW, Third Floor, Washington, DC 20001-2085
E-mail: books@cwla.org

CURRENT PRINTING (last digit)
10 9 8 7 6 5 4 3 2 1

Cover design by Luke Johnson

Printed in the United States of America

ISBN # 0–87868-749-1

Library of Congress Cataloging-in-Publication Data
Rahrer, J. Stuart
Seven sensible strategies for drug-free kids / J. Stuart Rahrer
p. cm.
Includes bibliographical references
ISBN 0-87868-749-1 (alk. paper)
1. Children--drug use--Prevention. 2. Children--Alcohol use--Prevention. 3. Drug abuse--Prevention. 4. Alcoholism--Prevention.
I. Title
HV5824.C45R395 1999 99-28331
649'.4--dc21 CIP

Contents

Acknowledgments

I want to thank Karen Asp for her invaluable editorial assistance. Her ideas and superb editing made this a much better book. Additionally, a special thanks is due to Susan Brite, the Director of Publications for the Child Welfare League of America, for her invaluable assistance in the overall production of this book. Her insight about the need for such a book, as well as her patience and perseverance, was important to me and much appreciated. I would also like to publicly thank the many other people, too numerous to mention, including various mental health professionals, educators, parents, grandparents, single parents, foster parents, and other child caregivers, who have been generous with their time and effort in providing input, suggestions, and editorial comments in the preparation of this book.

Disclaimer

Introduction

As a parent, protecting and helping your child become a productive, independent, and responsible person is one of your highest priorities, and this book will help you fulfill that responsibility. I have written this book to provide you with knowledge and a plan of action to prevent or stop your child's alcohol and other drug (AOD) abuse, regardless of whether you are a part of a two-parent family, a single parent, foster parent, adoptive parent, grandparent, or guardian. *Seven Sensible Strategies for Drug-Free Kids* is not only a book to read, but also a resource to use.

How It Works

Quick decisions based on answers to quizzes in magazines, newspapers, or television can cause fear, anxiety, and overreaction among parents and caregivers, often resulting in needless conflicts with their children. Similarly, advertisements stressing the terrible consequences of child AOD abuse appeal to the heart instead of the head. In some cases, these appeals only serve to recruit bewildered parents and caregivers for a free evaluation that may or may not be accurate or in the best interest of the child. Simple evaluations with easy solutions or 30-second commercials oversimplify complex issues and are misleading. Caregivers need to have a more in-depth approach and this book provides it. Here's how.

First, you will complete the Evaluation Inventory to detect and measure the extent of your child or teen's AOD use, as well as a questionnaire to identify high-risk factors for AOD abuse. Based on your answers, you will be given recommendations to use one of three strategies to prevent or stop your child's AOD abuse. The first two are prevention strategies, and both have a similar format. Strategy 1 is more appropriate for younger children ages 5 to 10, while Strategy 2 involves activities more suitable for older children. There is a possibility that you may use both prevention strategies, but the age of your child is the starting point. On the other hand, if there is evidence of an AOD problem or a high-risk factor, Strategy 3 will be recommended as your initial step.

Strategy 1. Determining If Your Child Is At Risk for AOD Abuse

Using Strategy 1, you will complete the 140-item At-Risk Inventory to determine if your child is at risk for AOD abuse. Then you will learn how to convert the identified at-risk characteristics into personal objectives for use in a prevention plan. This strategy is suitable for younger children.

Strategy 2. Designing a Personalized Plan to Prevent Your Child's AOD Abuse

Using Strategy 2, you will learn how to design and use your own individualized plan to maximize your efforts in preventing your child's AOD abuse. Your plan will be based on tasks and activities you select from the 115-item Prevention Inventory. This strategy is recommended for children older than 10 years.

Strategy 3. Consulting with a Professional to Determine If Your Child Has an AOD Problem

This strategy provides you with a Recommendation Worksheet to help you arrange a consultation with a professional to determine if your child has an AOD-related problem. The strategy includes suggestions about how to select a professional, as well as what to expect at the consultation. Based on the results of the consultation, you will learn how to make the best decision about your child's AOD situation. Your options include the following:

- If no AOD abuse or other serious problems exist and your child is between the ages of 5 and 10, you will use Strategy 1, Determining If Your Child Is At Risk for AOD Abuse.
- If no AOD abuse or other serious problems exist and your child is between the ages of 9 and 13, you will use Strategy 2, Designing a Personalized Plan to Prevent Your Child's AOD Abuse.
- If outpatient counseling is recommended, you will use Strategy 4, Knowing What to Expect from Outpatient Counseling.
- If a change in the home environment is recommended, you will use Strategy 5, Designing the Structured Home Environment: Expectations, Choices, and Consequences.
- If an intervention is recommended, you will use Strategy 6, Understanding How and When to Use the Intervention Process.
- If inpatient or residential treatment is recommended, you will use Strategy 7, Selecting an Effective Inpatient/Residential Treatment Program.

Strategy 4. Knowing What to Expect from Outpatient Counseling

Usually, the consulting professional will be the outpatient counselor. But if this is not the case, you'll be able to select a counselor using the criteria established in Strategy 3. You'll also learn what to expect from outpatient counseling and how you will be involved in the process.

Strategy 5. Designing the Structured Home Environment: Expectations, Choices, and Consequences

This strategy will show you how to implement a ten-step process to make your child more accountable and responsible for her behavior. You will discover what to expect from your child when using this structure and how to respond. You will also learn what to do if your child continues abusing AOD.

Strategy 6. Understanding How and When to Use the Intervention Process

If your child does not respond to prevention measures, a structured home environment, or professional counseling efforts, intervention may be necessary to get your child in touch with the reality of his condition and the need for help. Using this strategy, you will learn how the intervention process works and how to do it, step by step.

Strategy 7. Selecting an Effective Inpatient/Residential Treatment Program

If your child is out of control, almost dysfunctional and risking his life and the lives of others by abusing AOD, the last alternative is commitment to an inpatient or residential treatment program. This strategy offers a Selection Workshop to help you select the best treatment facility to meet your family's needs and discover what to expect before, during, and after treatment.

Your child's needs and choices will determine which of the strategies you will use. *You* are in charge of the situation, however, and this book is your guide as it takes you through strategies that are intertwined into a proactive plan. In the end, this sensible plan of action will dramatically increase your prospects of success in preventing or stopping your child's AOD abuse.

A Final Word

After 25 years of working with childhood and adolescent AOD-related problems, I realize two important factors. One is that *listening* has been the greatest source of my information and wisdom: Listening to countless numbers of parents, grandparents, and foster parents share their experiences about their children and about their successes, failures, frustrations, and joys. I am deeply grateful for the education they have given me. Secondly, I am aware of how painfully uninformed I still am about these issues. I learn and continue to grow each day. With that in mind, I want you to know this book is not intended to be the last word on the subject. I anticipate a future revised edition filled with additional input from parents and caregivers. Please feel free to share your experiences and suggestions, so that I can make this book better for the parents and caregivers of tomorrow. I enthusiastically look forward to my ongoing education and growth.

Detecting Child or Adolescent AOD Use

You think your child would never use alcohol or other drugs (AOD), but you're not sure. You read and hear about the terrible things happening with young people and AOD abuse... but your child? No way! Well, maybe. Who knows?

Unfortunately, parents and caregivers must face this dilemma, because they are not certain that their child would use AOD, but they are curious to find out. Of course, parents and caregivers must also be careful not to upset family harmony and stability in doing so. If this is you, you have a solution in hand.

This chapter provides you with a working knowledge about addiction and the process of acquiring an addiction. (This information will help you understand the stages of AOD use that will be discussed later.) Then you will complete the easy-to-follow, 120-question Evaluation Inventory of your child's AOD use. You will also complete a questionnaire to determine if your child is currently at high risk for AOD abuse. The purpose is to detect and measure the extent of your child or teen's AOD use and identify high-risk factors. Based on these results, you will be given a recommendation to use one of three strategies.

An *addiction* is the repeated use of an object (AOD) or behavior for a reward that a person cannot or will not stop despite the negative consequences. Regardless of age, gender, race, socioeconomic status, or religion, millions of people develop addictions. The four-stage pattern of addiction depicted in the detection evaluation below will help you better understand the sequence of symptoms. The reason an addiction develops is rooted in a perplexing and powerfully driven process that significantly alters how a person thinks and behaves. This thought and behavior pattern is generally misunderstood and mistaken by many as a lack of will-power, moral degeneracy, or just plain insanity.

The Addiction Process

Listed below are two terms frequently used in discussions of the addiction process:

- **Agent.** The object used by the person. Examples of AOD objects include alcohol; tobacco; prescribed medications; inhalants; over-the-counter cough, cold, sleep, and diet medications; marijuana; cocaine or crack; LSD; PCP; opiates; heroin; and "designer drugs."

- **Reward.** Any immediate, temporary mood change or gratification caused by the use of AOD.

The addiction process is initiated by the *repeated* use of an AOD agent to get an immediate reward. The reward, or the mood change—not the AOD—gets the person's attention. Thereafter, the reward becomes the alluring and seductive "hook" in the process. This is the reason why the behavior is repeated and valued. The person learns, by accident or design, that AOD can provide a reward or mood change, such as feelings of relief, escape, or confidence.

The use of AOD can temporarily lessen or seemingly eliminate moods and feelings of anxiety, boredom, confusion, depression, failure, guilt or shame, inadequacy, loneliness, hopelessness, rejection, or stress.

The repeated use of AOD to get the reward becomes compulsive. The person obsessively thinks about AOD and plans for the next reward to feel better. He repeatedly seeks out and uses AOD to get the reward and experiences an irresistible urge to use AOD in an excessive or irrational way.

Thinking about AOD and the reward consumes the person's time, energy, and attention. He often feels anxious or excited before receiving the reward from AOD and gets upset, frustrated, or panicked if something interferes with the performance of AOD. Often, the *anticipation* of use is more consuming than the *actual* use of AOD. Thoughts and preoccupation about how, when, and where to use AOD structure and organize his day, and the relationship between AOD and the reward becomes more valuable than anyone or anything in his life.

After a period of time, a loss of control becomes evident. The person cannot or will not stop the behavior, nor recognize it as a problem, despite the unpleasant, painful, or destructive consequences that occur in one or more areas of his life, including personal, social, recreational, and academic or professional functions and relationships; mental, psychological, spiritual, and physical health; and/or judgment and finances.

To defend the continued use of AOD and get the reward, the person develops a host of strategies to deny that the use of AOD has anything to do with his problems. The strategies include *minimizing* ("It's no big deal." "It's not that bad."); *avoiding the subject* (ignoring or refusing to talk about it or distracting others from the subject); *absolute denying* ("I can stop anytime." "No, I don't have a problem." "I'm not as bad as Elvis was." "How can a behavior be addicting?") and *blaming others* ("My parents and caregivers, friends, and teachers are driving me nuts." "Yes, I do it, but so would anybody in my situation.")

At this point, the addiction process has been completed and the person is *addicted* to the reward provided by AOD, despite the terrible consequences of using the AOD. Initially, AOD produced the rewards of pleasure, relief, a sense of control, and other payoffs. The short-term benefits are eventually overtaken by the negative effects of the use of AOD, however. The reward has now become so dependable and valued by the person that he constantly pursues AOD to get the reward. The reward is valued above and beyond anyone and anything else and the person's life becomes a pursuit of the reward to provide a sense of control in his out-of-control life.

The Evaluation Inventory

The following evaluation inventory is based on extensive research conducted to identify specific child attitudinal, behavioral, and physical symptoms of AOD abuse. The symptoms have been identified and arranged in a sequence most likely to occur. Not every young person will experience each symptom, nor will the symptoms occur in an exact sequence. In addition, they may or may not be the direct result of AOD abuse. The number, location, and consistency of your responses will reveal a pattern that will determine and measure the extent and possibility of AOD use.

Instructions

Note: The inventory is not to be used for clinical assessment or diagnosis unless under the direction and supervision of a qualified professional. It is solely intended to help you as a parent or caregiver determine whether or not you have a potential AOD abuse problem with your child and what to do about it.

Because you may want to use this book again or share it with others, copy and use the Answer Sheet on page 18. To complete the evaluation inventory, respond to each of the items by selecting an answer according to what you have observed, thought, or felt about your child's attitude, behavior, or physical characteristics with the following scale:

N = No
Y = Yes
S = Seldom
F = Frequently
? = Don't Know

With certain items, the responses are

N = No
Y = Yes
? = Don't Know

Stage 1. Experimental Use

This stage typically begins during late elementary and junior high school. The child may try AOD once or twice because she is curious about the effects or has a natural desire to experiment. In wanting to feel grown up, she may also be influenced by peer group appeal. The major activities include drinking alcohol, smoking pot or cigarettes, or sniffing glue. These activities may occur at home, at a party, or while hanging out with friends. Small amounts of AOD are needed to get high, and the child usually returns to a normal mood without complications. The child has learned to use AOD to alter her mood and the pleasure centers of the brain, however. Most young people believe that what feels good must be good, and few think they will ever die from engaging in what feels good. In this case, curiosity and experimentation, coupled with feelings of immortality, can prove to be dangerous.

To determine if your child may have experimented with drugs, answer the following questions, using the Answer Sheet on page 18.

1. Do you think your child has used any AOD, not including nicotine or caffeine?
2. Do you think your child has used AOD in the last six months?
3. Do you think your child has used AOD during the past three months?
4. Does she have low self-esteem?
5. Is your child impatient and easily frustrated?
6. Does he volunteer to clean up after a cocktail party that you host?
7. Has your liquor supply mysteriously disappeared?
8. Are there mysterious phone calls made to or by your child?
9. Have you noticed that you have run out of prescription medications sooner than expected?
10. Does your child defy your authority?
11. Is your child irresponsible about household chores?
12. Is your child disrespectful or critical of your life style?
13. Does she show less interest in family leisure and recreational activities?
14. Does he avoid conversation with family members most of the time?

15. Does your child request extra money for lunch, school supplies, etc.?
16. Does your child show less interest in school?
17. Does she have discipline problems with teachers and other school officials?
18. Has he changed friends recently?
19. Does your child party with the new friends?
20. Are her new friends older, use hip jargon, and possibly use AOD?
21. When new friends visit, do they immediately go to your child's room, close the door and turn on the music?
22. Does he listen to rap, acid, heavy metal, or rock music and decorate his room with psychedelic posters or colors?
23. Does she quickly leave home after a phone call without an explanation?
24. Has he shown a distinct, unusual personality or mood change?
25. Does she tell obvious and unnecessary lies?
26. Does he tune out if or when AOD are discussed?
27. Does she spend much time alone in her room?
28. Does he burn incense in his room?
29. Does she excessively use breath mints, possibly masking the smell of alcohol?
30. Have you noticed a peculiar odor on your child or her clothes, such as the smell of burning rope?
31. Has your child started using cigarettes?
32. Have you smelled alcohol on your child's breath?

Stage 2. Occasional and Increasing Use

During this stage, AOD use begins to increase. The child may progress to hard liquor and increase AOD use to get drunk, catch a buzz, or get high with peers at social activities. Because the abuse of AOD may become related to dealing with stress, the child begins to abuse during the week. By now, the body has developed tolerance and more problems begin to occur, such as missing school because of hangovers, missing time on a job, or not performing well in sports. The child may even try different drugs, including hallucinogens and pills. Friends who don't use AOD may be forgotten as new, older friends appear. More money may be needed, leading to stealing from family as well as lying to hide AOD use. The child's moods may change rapidly without explanation and interest in usual activities may dwindle. You may have noticed these changes in your child. The following questions will help you confirm these changes.

33. Does her pattern of use reflect more than 12 Yes responses from Stage 1?
34. Has he used AOD for more than one year?
35. Do you think your child has used AOD more than two times during the past month?
36. Have you found empty liquor bottles, pipes, hair clips, cigarette papers, or other drug paraphernalia in her room?
37. Have his school grades declined?
38. Has your child quit extracurricular activities?
39. Has your child stopped associating with old friends?
40. Does she vehemently try to convince you that she has no drinking or drug problem?
41. Have you noticed a mysterious disappearance of valuables or money, maybe payment for AOD?
42. Is he often late for home, school, or job?
43. Is your child often absent from school?
44. Does your child fail to come home at a specific time?
45. Does your child have a runny nose or bloodshot eyes without having a cold, allergy, or the flu?
46. Do more than 25% of her friends use AOD?

47. Have his old friends stopped associating with him?
48. Does your child belligerently defend her new friends and the right to drink and use marijuana?
49. Has your child hidden liquor or drug paraphernalia?
50. Has he become increasingly dishonest?
51. Has your child developed poor, irregular eating habits?
52. Are your child's sleeping habits irregular or does she have insomnia?
53. Does he isolate himself?
54. Does she laugh for no apparent reason?
55. Does he appear unusually disheveled or unkempt?
56. Does she have periodic mood swings between use?
57. Is your child unreliable and unpredictable?
58. Have her personal hygiene habits drastically declined?
59. Do you think he uses AOD during the week?
60. Does your child use more than one drug, excluding nicotine and caffeine?
61. Is there evidence of burns on her fingers, clothing, furniture, or rugs, possibly from handling things when high?
62. Does your child have a bad attitude in the morning from a possible hangover, depression, or low self-esteem?
63. Has he spent unexplained or unusual amounts of money?
64. Does your child wear sunglasses and have sensitive eyes?
65. Are her eye pupils abnormally dilated or constricted occasionally?
66. Does he wear sunglasses to cover dilated, constricted, or bloodshot eyes?
67. If old enough, has your teen refused to look for part-time work or been unable to hold a job?
68. Is he hyperactive?
69. Is she listless?
70. Has your teen dropped out of school?
71. Has your child fought with peers?

Stage 3. Regular Use and Daily Preoccupation with the Mood Swing

This stage usually develops during the adolescent years as AOD abuse increases and the effects become more evident. The teen begins to use on a regular basis and attempts normal behavior and activities at home, school, and with peers. Often, more dangerous drugs are used, causing additional problems in significant areas of the teen's life. AOD abuse becomes a central focus of life, and the teen thinks about the last high and when, with whom, and where the next high will take place. The preoccupation with AOD abuse begins to replace thoughts of and activities with family, school, and community. In addition, more critical problems develop that often involve stealing, breaking laws, and participating in violence. As guilt, shame, loneliness, and depression (partially concealed by denial and grandiosity) set in due to withdrawal from or cravings for AOD, mood changes occur. The teen attempts to cut down or quit but is usually unsuccessful. Serious physical problems may also begin to develop.

Use the following questions to determine if AOD use has increased.

72. Does your teen's pattern of use reflect more than 12 Yes responses in Stage 1 and more than 10 Yes responses in Stage 2?
73. Has she experienced significant negative consequences after using AOD?
74. Does he use AOD to cope with stress and feelings?
75. Has she continued to use AOD after significant consequences, such as vomiting, grounding, or getting into accidents?
76. Is there evidence of a pattern of AOD use that includes binge drinking and regular weekend use?
77. Does he use AOD in physically hazardous situations?
78. Does she use breath mints throughout the day?
79. Have you noticed obvious hangovers with headaches and nausea?
80. Is she aggressive, uptight, and paranoid?
81. Have friends and neighbors made comments about his behavior?
82. Have her important social, occupational, and recreational activities declined because of her use of AOD?
83. Do his behaviors now include stealing, lying, and arguing with family members?

84. Does she have extreme mood swings?
85. Is his nose red and raw?
86. Have there been more than four AOD-related incidents in the past six months?
87. Does she show unusual hyperactivity or slurred speech?
88. Does your teen hang out in known drug locations?
89. Has he been associating with known AOD users?
90. Has she been involved in dealing drugs to others?
91. Has your teen made attempts to cut down or quit AOD?
92. Have her consequences included driving while intoxicated on one occasion or an arrest for a motor vehicle accident within the past six months?
93. Is he unable to maintain a no-AOD-use contract for 30 days?
94. Has her longest period of abstinence in the past six months been less than one week?

Stage 4. Chronic Use and Harmful Dependency

This stage often involves more dangerous drugs in larger amounts. Because the teen is surrounded by AOD-using peers and situations, he no longer understands normal behavior. His AOD abuse is out of control and life has become unmanageable in many areas, including physical, psychological, social, family, school, and legal situations. The teen feels guilt, shame, and self-hatred, which sometimes lead to suicidal thoughts and attempts. Because of physical tolerance, the teen no longer gets as high, and much more time is spent attempting to get relief, trying to feel normal, and avoiding withdrawal symptoms. He experiences severe physical, social, and emotional consequences and uses AOD to relieve the pain and unpleasantness caused by his addiction. This vicious circle will continue until he quits using AOD and a subsequent commitment is made to recover from the addiction. To determine if your child is dependent on AOD, answer these questions:

95. Does your teen's pattern of use reflect more than 12 Yes responses in Stage 1, more than 10 Yes responses in Stage 2, and more than 2 Yes responses in Stage 3?
96. Has your teen shown pronounced irrational behavior or made dangerous threats?
97. Does your teen have pronounced guilty feelings or paranoia?
98. Does he appear irrational or delusional?
99. Is there evidence of significant depression, suicidal thoughts, or self-destructive behavior?
100. Has your teen suddenly lost weight?
101. Does she pass out in her room or appear in a semiconscious state?
102. Has there been an increased frequency in his drinking and drugging episodes, blackouts, and erratic behavior?
103. Has your family life generally deteriorated and become fragmented?
104. Has your teen received professional counseling for behavioral problems?
105. Does her preoccupation with AOD or intoxication consistently interfere with her obligations?
106. Does he use AOD daily?
107. Does she use AOD in the morning?

108. Have you noticed his hands shaking or trembling in the morning?

109. Has your teen been arrested for shoplifting, trespassing, using, or possessing AOD more than once?

110. Has your teen been arrested for drunk driving more than once?

111. Does she have burns or scorch marks on nose, lips, or face?

112. Does he sweat profusely, even on cold days?

113. Does she have swollen and puffy hands or feet?

114. Have you noticed your teen constantly sniffling?

115. Have you found burned spoons or bottle caps?

116. Have you found knotted shoestrings or pantyhose that may have been used as an arm tie for intravenous use?

117. Does he wear long-sleeved shirts in warm weather?

118. Have you noticed track or needle marks on her arms, hands, legs, or neck?

119. Has he admitted to daily AOD use and preoccupation with chemicals?

120. Does your teen have:

- Ulcers?
- AIDS?
- Liver problems?
- Kidney disorders?
- Chronic indigestion?
- Pneumonia?
- Gastritis?
- Bronchitis?
- Depression?
- Suicidal thoughts?

Scoring

Now refer to each of the four stages and count the numbers of the N, Y, S, F, and ? responses separately. Then add the totals and place your scores in the box below.

Stage 1	Stage 2	Stage 3	Stage 4	Totals
N ______	N ______	N ______	N ______	N ______
Y ______	Y ______	Y ______	Y ______	Y ______
S ______	S ______	S ______	S ______	S ______
F ______	F ______	F ______	F ______	F ______
? ______	? ______	? ______	? ______	? ______

Analysis and Follow-Up

Before you begin scoring, please remember that this evaluation inventory is not to be used for a *clinical assessment* or *diagnosis* unless under the direction and supervision of a qualified professional. It is intended *solely* to help you determine if you have a potential AOD abuse problem with your child and what to do about it. Your options will include prevention efforts, continued monitoring, or consultation with a mental health professional.

Answers will vary among parents and caregivers, depending on the different characteristics of each child. Moreover, the symptoms do not necessarily occur in the sequence presented in the evaluation and may or may not be the direct result of AOD abuse. The intent of the inventory is to determine the number, location, and consistency of your responses to reveal a pattern that most likely determines and measures the extent and possibility of AOD abuse.

Now, review your responses and make sure you have accurately answered each item. Then refer to the following section, "Options You Have."

Options You Have

Interpretation/Indicators/Recommendations

Yes (Y) and Frequently (F) answers are red flag responses. A number of these responses in any stage should receive careful consideration in the interpretation and recommendation process.

No (N) and Seldom (S) answers are favorable responses. They should be reviewed periodically, however, to see if the S responses have changed to F incidents or situations.

Don't Know (?) answers are just that. They may or may not signal trouble in the future. To find out, be aware of the items and continue to monitor these responses periodically.

Stage 1: Experimental Use

Interpretation #1

- Less than 12 Y and F responses in Stage 1
- Less than 10 Y and F responses in Stage 2
- No more than two Y and F responses in Stage 3
- No more than two Y and F responses in Stage 4

If you have all of the above requirements, there is little evidence to suggest a potential AOD abuse problem at this time. Your child may be at high risk for developing a problem, however. If so, this may require a different strategy. To make sure, complete the questionnaire on page 16, "High-Risk Factors for AOD Abuse."

Interpretation #2

If your Y and F responses totaled 11 or more in Stage 1, there may be a pattern leading into occasional AOD use. Continue to monitor your child and carefully review your responses in Stage 2.

Interpretation #3

It is possible to overlook or not observe certain characteristics in Stages 1 and 2. Therefore, if you have less than 12 F responses in Stage 1, but more than 10 F responses in Stage 2 or more than two F responses in Stage 3 or 4, arrange for a consultation with a mental health professional by using Strategy 3, especially if your F responses total five or more in either Stages 3 or 4.

Stage 2: Occasional and Increasing Use

Interpretation #1

- More than 12 Y and F responses in Stage 1
- Less than 10 Y and F responses in Stage 2
- No more than two Y and F responses in Stage 3
- No more than two Y and F responses in Stage 4

If you have all of the above requirements, there is little evidence to suggest a potential AOD abuse problem at this time. Your child may be at high-risk for developing a problem, however. If so, this may require a different strategy. To make sure, complete the questionnaire on page 16, "High-Risk Factors for AOD Abuse."

Interpretation #2

If your Y and F responses totaled 11 or more in Stage 1, there may be a pattern leading into occasional AOD use. Continue to monitor your child and carefully review your responses in Stage 2.

Interpretation #3

It is possible to overlook or not observe certain characteristics in Stages 1 and 2. Therefore, if you have less than 12 F responses in Stage 1 and less than 10 F responses in Stage 2, but more than two F responses in Stage 3 or 4, arrange for a consultation with a mental health professional, especially if you have five or more F responses in either Stages 3 or 4.

Interpretation #4

- More than 12 Y and F responses in Stage 1
- More than 10 Y and F responses in Stage 2
- No more than two Y and F responses in Stage 3
- No more than two Y and F responses in Stage 4

If you have all of the above requirements, the possibility of occasional to regular AOD abuse exists. Arrange for a consultation with a mental health professional, especially if you have five or more F responses in either Stages 3 or 4.

Stage 3: Regular Use and Daily Preoccupation with the Mood Swing

Interpretation #1

- More than 12 Y and F responses in Stage 1
- More than 10 Y and F responses in Stage 2
- At least two Y and F responses in Stage 3
- No more than two Y and F responses in Stage 4

If you have all of the above requirements, there is a strong possibility of regular AOD abuse. Arrange for a consultation with a mental health professional, especially if your F responses total five or more in either Stages 3 or 4. As previously noted, the symptoms in the evaluation do not necessarily occur in the exact sequence presented and may or may not be the direct result of AOD abuse. This dilemma can be resolved during your session with a mental health professional who has expertise in treating addictions and chemical dependency.

Stage 4: Chronic Use and Harmful Dependency

Interpretation #1

- More than 12 Y and F responses in Stage 1
- More than 10 Y and F responses in Stage 2
- More than two Y and F responses in Stage 3
- More than two Y and F responses in Stage 4

If you have all of the above requirements, there is a probability of AOD dependency with harmful consequences. Arrange for a consultation with a mental health professional, especially if your F responses total five or more in either Stages 3 or 4.

Question 120

If you responded YES to any of the physical or emotional problems listed under this question, review the results of the evaluation with your family physician. If there is a possible link to the physical or emotional problems and AOD abuse, refer to Strategy 3 beginning on page 61 and follow the procedure to arrange a consultation with a mental health professional.

Regardless of your score, read as much material about the subject (turn to the recommended reading list and bibliography at the back of this book for suggestions), learn as much as possible about child and teen AOD abuse, and tailor the information to your needs.

High-Risk Factors for AOD Abuse

To determine if your child is at high risk for AOD abuse, respond to the following statements:

- Your child is rebellious and feels alienated. True/False
- Your child has shown early antisocial behavior. True/False
- Your child has experienced early, heavy AOD use. True/False
- Your child has a low interest in school and adult achievement. True/False
- Your child is a school dropout. True/False
- Your child has experienced repeated failure in school. True/False
- Your child has become pregnant. True/False
- Your child is economically disadvantaged. True/False
- Your child is the child of an AOD abuser. True/False
- Your child is a victim of physical, sexual, or psychological abuse. True/False
- Your child has committed a violent or delinquent act. True/False
- Your child has experienced mental health problems. True/False
- Your child has attempted suicide. True/False
- Your child deals drugs to make money. True/False
- Your child has been arrested for delinquent behavior. True/False

Recommendations

If you answered *false* to all of the statements, your child is presently not at high risk for AOD abuse. Therefore, select one of the following prevention strategies that is appropriate for your child:

- If your child is between the ages of 5 and 10, refer to Strategy 1 on page 19. This strategy is typically more appropriate for younger children, but consider using Strategy 2 as well. Although Strategy 2 is more suitable for children over age 10, you may find that it also applies to your situation.
- If your child is older than 10, refer to Strategy 2 on page 41, but consider using Strategy 1 as well. Although Strategy 1 is more suitable for younger children, you may find that it also applies to your situation.

- If you answered *true* to no more than two of the statements, your child may not presently be at high risk for AOD abuse. Take into account the seriousness of each high-risk factor, however, monitor the situation, and consider using Strategy 3 if the situation does not improve. In the meantime, select one of the prevention strategies described above that is appropriate for your child.
- If you answered *true* to at least three or more of these statements, there is an indication of a high risk for AOD abuse. This doesn't mean that your child has an AOD-related problem. Rather, it represents a warning sign that you should check out with a professional. In this case, refer to Strategy 3 on page 61. This section describes how to select and arrange a consultation with a mental health professional to discover if your child has an AOD problem. Take the results of your evaluation and questionnaire to the professional consultant. The information will be helpful.

Intuition

You should now have enough information to determine if your child abuses AOD. You are also in a position to take action by following the recommendations based on your specific results. There is just one exception. Over the years, I have developed an abiding faith in intuition—the gut feeling that something is wrong with your child. If you have that feeling, regardless of what you have read or what others have told you, arrange a consultation with a mental health professional. The professional will help you sort out your feelings and observations to help you determine what is best for your child. It will be one of the best investments you could ever make.

Answer Sheet

Stage 1

1. N Y S F ?
2. N Y S F ?
3. N Y S F ?
4. N Y S F ?
5. N Y S F ?
6. N Y S F ?
7. N Y S F ?
8. N Y S F ?
9. N Y S F ?
10. N Y S F ?
11. N Y S F ?
12. N Y S F ?
13. N Y S F ?
14. N Y S F ?
15. N Y S F ?
16. N Y S F ?
17. N Y S F ?
18. N Y S F ?
19. N Y S F ?
20. N Y S F ?
21. N Y S F ?
22. N Y S F ?
23. N Y S F ?
24. N Y S F ?
25. N Y S F ?
26. N Y S F ?
27. N Y S F ?
28. N Y S F ?
29. N Y S F ?
30. N Y S F ?
31. N Y S F ?
32. N Y S F ?

Stage 2

33. N Y S F ?
34. N Y S F ?
35. N Y S F ?
36. N Y S F ?
37. N Y S F ?
38. N Y S F ?
39. N Y S F ?
40. N Y S F ?
41. N Y S F ?
42. N Y S F ?
43. N Y S F ?
44. N Y S F ?
45. N Y S F ?
46. N Y S F ?
47. N Y S F ?
48. N Y S F ?
49. N Y S F ?
50. N Y S F ?
51. N Y S F ?
52. N Y S F ?
53. N Y S F ?
54. N Y S F ?
55. N Y S F ?
56. N Y S F ?
57. N Y S F ?
58. N Y S F ?
59. N Y S F ?
60. N Y S F ?
61. N Y S F ?
62. N Y S F ?
63. N Y S F ?
64. N Y S F ?
65. N Y S F ?
66. N Y S F ?
67. N Y S F ?
68. N Y S F ?
69. N Y S F ?
70. N Y S F ?
71. N Y S F ?

Stage 3

72. N Y S F ?
73. N Y S F ?
74. N Y S F ?
75. N Y S F ?
76. N Y S F ?
77. N Y S F ?
78. N Y S F ?
79. N Y S F ?
80. N Y S F ?
81. N Y S F ?
82. N Y S F ?
83. N Y S F ?
84. N Y S F ?
85. N Y S F ?
86. N Y S F ?
87. N Y S F ?
88. N Y S F ?
89. N Y S F ?
90. N Y S F ?
91. N Y S F ?
92. N Y S F ?
93. N Y S F ?
94. N Y S F ?

Stage 4

95. N Y S F ?
96. N Y S F ?
97. N Y S F ?
98. N Y S F ?
99. N Y S F ?
100. N Y S F ?
101. N Y S F ?
102. N Y S F ?
103. N Y S F ?
104. N Y S F ?
105. N Y S F ?
106. N Y S F ?
107. N Y S F ?
108. N Y S F ?
109. N Y S F ?
110. N Y S F ?
111. N Y S F ?
112. N Y S F ?
113. N Y S F ?
114. N Y S F ?
115. N Y S F ?
116. N Y S F ?
117. N Y S F ?
118. N Y S F ?
119. N Y S F ?
120. See page 115.

Strategy 1

Determining If Your Child Is At Risk for AOD Abuse

Most children are curious enough to experiment with alcohol or other drugs (AOD) and then stop. Some continue to use incidentally without any significant problems, while others use on a regular basis and experience varying degrees of physical, emotional, and social consequences. Sadly, some of these children develop a self-destructive AOD abuse pattern and become an emotional, social, and costly burden to significant others and society. AOD abusers can die; their actions can also lead to the deaths of others.

It is difficult to say where your child will fit into this scenario if you do nothing about his potential AOD abuse. But you can start protecting your child now by using this strategy to determine if your child is at risk for AOD abuse. Strategy 1 provides you with the 140-item At-Risk Inventory to determine if your child is at risk for AOD abuse. You will learn how to convert the identified at-risk characteristics into personal objectives that you will use in a prevention plan. Before starting the inventory, you will be given an overview of the extent of AOD use among young people, based on current surveys and statistics. This will give you an idea of the situation your child has witnessed and the formidable challenge you face. Next, you will complete the inventory by answering each of the 140 items.

Once you have completed the At-Risk Inventory, you will list your responses on three separate worksheets. Then you will be shown how to convert your responses into prevention objectives that you will place on a master sheet. Next, you will assign a priority value and completion date for each objective. At the end of the process, you will have up to 140 objectives to help prevent your child's AOD abuse. If the strategy is successful, you will be encouraged to consider Strategy 2 for additional information, which has a number of possible prevention objectives that you may decide to use on your master sheet. Use the evaluation instrument on a periodic basis. If you detect AOD abuse and a consultation with a professional is recommended, use Strategy 3 on page 61.

The Extent of Child AOD Abuse: What You and Your Child Are Facing

To give you an idea of what you are facing, take a look at a random sampling of recent surveys and statistics dealing with child AOD use. The National Parents' Resource Institute for Drug Education (PRIDE) conducted a study during the 1994-95 school year that involved 198,241 students in 32 states from California to New York. Participating schools received the PRIDE questionnaire with explicit instructions for administering the anonymous survey. The schools participated on a voluntary basis or in compliance with a school district or state request. The results, which were released in November 1995 represented data from sixth through twelfth grade students [PRIDE, no date], which led to the following conclusions:

- In recent years, marijuana use increased more dramatically than any other drug in the study. One-third of high school seniors (33%) smoked marijuana in the past year, and more than one-fifth (21%) smoked monthly.
- There were significant increases in cigarette and marijuana use by students in grades 6 through 12 during the 1994-95 school year. Students in grades 9 through 12 also reported increases in cocaine and hallucinogen use.
- In high school (grades 9 through 12), cocaine and hallucinogen use increased annually and monthly.
- Beer drinking by high school students reached a five-year high and in junior high, a two-year high.
- One in three high school seniors smoked marijuana.
- Since the 1990-91 school year, annual reported use of marijuana in junior high school (grades 6 through 8) has risen 111% (from 4.5% to 9.5%) and 67% in high school (16.9% vs. 28.2%).
- The so-called "hard drugs," cocaine and hallucinogens, reached their highest levels of use among high school students since the 1988-89 school year. There was a 36% increase (from 3% to 4.5%) in cocaine use by students in grades 9 through 12 since 1991-92, the period of lowest use in recent years. Hallucinogen use had risen 75% (from 4.4% to 7.7%) since 1988-89, the recent low point.
- In the eight years of the PRIDE national survey, cigarette use reached its highest levels during the 1994-95 school year. Nearly half (44%) of high school students smoked at least once in the past year, compared with 37% in 1988-89. In grades 6 through 12, nearly one-third (28%) of students smoked.

Another study prepared in 1995 for the New York-based Partnership for a Drug-Free America surveyed the practices and attitudes of 12,292 children, teens and parents and found the following [Partnership for a Drug-Free America, no date]:

- Kids are beginning to use drugs, especially marijuana, at a younger age than ever before. Marijuana use by youngsters in grades 4-6 has doubled.
- Among the findings for kids ages 9 to 12:
  - The trial use of marijuana increased from 2% to 4% between 1993 and 1994, which represents an increase from about 230,000 to 450,000 children experimenting with marijuana.
  - The percentage of white children who agreed with the statement, "Everybody tries drugs," increased from 21% to 28% in 1995.
  - Fewer children than in previous surveys said they would tell their parents if someone offered them drugs.
  - One out of every four children was offered drugs in 1993.
  - The number of youngsters ages 11 and 12 who said they have friends using marijuana increased from 7% to 13%.*

Additionally, the tenth annual PRIDE Survey for the school year 1996-97 (released on October 28, 1997), which involved 141,077 students in junior and senior high schools from 28 states, revealed the following:

- Students in junior high (grades 6-8) reported statistically significant increases in monthly use of marijuana, cocaine, uppers, downers, hallucinogens, and heroin. One-tenth (11%) of junior high students, mostly ages 11-14, were current (monthly) drug users.
- One-quarter of senior high students (25%) used an illicit drug on a monthly or more frequent basis in the past school year. Seven percent said they took illegal drugs daily, a figure that rose to 8% for the twelfth grade.
- More students (48%) said they attend parties "often" or "a lot" more than church (46%), and 15% said that they are likely to use drugs or alcohol at parties.
- Students were twice as likely to smoke marijuana at home than at school (13.5% vs. 6.5%) and more than four times more likely to smoke pot at a friend's house than at school (28.5% vs. 6.5%).

---

* The Partnership for a Drug-Free America survey was funded by the Robert Wood Johnson Foundation and was conducted by Audits and Surveys Worldwide, Inc. The 1995 Partnership Attitude Tracking Study (PATS) surveyed 9,342 people (6,096 teens, 2,424 preteens, and 822 parents). For a copy of the report, contact Partnership for a Drug-Free America at 405 Lexington Avenue, New York, NY 10174 or 212/922-1560.

- Use of two deadly, legal drugs (alcohol and nicotine from cigarettes) showed no abatement. Monthly cigarette smoking rose to 35% among high school students, while monthly use of hard liquor rose to 29% [PRIDE 1997].

These statistics make it clear. Young people are using AOD in dramatically increasing numbers and at younger ages. This is the reality of what you are facing and what your child is exposed to every day. By using this strategy, however, you will be able to identify and reduce the risks of your child's involvement with AOD.

The At-Risk Inventory

Your child is, has been, or will be exposed to distinct conditions and situations that may place her at risk for AOD abuse. She may also have specific physical, attitudinal, and behavioral traits (including certain psychological, social, biological, and spiritual features) that may qualify as at-risk characteristics. This combination of *characteristics* has been incorporated into the following At-Risk Inventory (ARI).

The inventory is based on extensive research and statistical analysis of the at-risk factors for child or teen AOD use. From the research findings, 140 items have been identified and selected for the ARI. The at-risk items, or characteristics, listed in the ARI should not be confused with symptoms of AOD abuse. Additionally, the inventory is not intended to predict if your child will abuse AOD or reveal that she has an addictive personality predisposing her to an addiction. Thus, it should not be used for clinical assessment or diagnosis unless under the direction and supervision of a qualified professional. The sole purpose is to help you identify your child's AOD at-risk characteristics and convert them into prevention objectives.

The at-risk characteristics of child AOD abuse have been divided into seven categories. Although each category is distinct, the characteristics in the categories are not mutually exclusive and often interact with one another:

- Genetic at-risk characteristics
- Pregnancy at-risk characteristics
- Individual personality and behavioral at-risk characteristics
- Home environment at-risk characteristics
- School at-risk characteristics
- Peer at-risk characteristics
- Community at-risk characteristics

Instructions

Respond to the items according to the following scale:

F = False
T = True
ST = Seldom True
OT = Often True
? = Don't Know

With certain items, the responses are only:

F = False
T = True
? = Don't Know

Please take time to consider your response to each item. Because you may want to use this book again or share it with others, copy and use the At-Risk Inventory Answer Sheet that is on page 40. When you have completed the ARI, refer to the section on page 34, "Identification and Selection of Prevention Objectives for Your Child."

Genetic At-Risk Characteristics

Although the biology and exact causes of AOD abuse remain a mystery, research indicates that there *may be* a genetic link to some kinds for AOD dependence. This means that some children could be more at risk to AOD abuse because of hereditary factors. Listed below are the clues to help you identify this potential tie-in.

1. Is your child adopted?
2. Did your child's biological father develop a problem with AOD and have delinquency and antisocial problems?
3. Did two or more biological male grandparents or uncles of your child ever have a problem with AOD (including prescription mind-altering drugs) and antisocial behavior?
4. Did your child's biological mother have AOD problems, including prescription medication abuse or overuse, an eating disorder, or somatic complaints?
5. Is your child primarily of Northern European ancestry?
6. Is your child primarily of Native American or Eskimo ancestry?

Pregnancy At-Risk Characteristics

AOD carried through the mother's bloodstream to her unborn child may cause a number of problems before, during, and after birth:

- **Alcohol.** Low birthweight and short length, small head size, facial defects, learning and behavioral problems
- **Cocaine.** More crying than normal, death before or after birth, less growth than normal, difficulty eating and sleeping
- **Tobacco.** Low weight at birth, death before birth, premature birth
- **Marijuana.** Death before birth or at birth, birth too early, low weight at birth
- **Crack.** Small head size, less growth than normal, learning problems, more crying than normal, difficulty eating and sleeping
- **Heroin.** Low weight at birth, more crying than normal, difficulty eating and sleeping, death at birth
- **PCP and LSD**. Death before birth, behavioral problems as the child gets older

7. Did your child's mother smoke heavily during the pregnancy?
8. Did your child's mother drink heavily during the entire pregnancy?
9. Did your child's mother use amphetamines, diet pills (even if prescribed by a physician), cocaine, or any type of speed during the pregnancy?

Individual Personality and Behavioral At-Risk Characteristics

Certain interrelated personality and behavioral characteristics have been identified and associated with a high risk of AOD problems among children. Children with a number of these characteristics are especially vulnerable to AOD abuse.

10. My child has a low self-esteem.
11. My child has little self-confidence, feels inadequate and incapable.
12. My child lacks self-identity.
13. My child is too self-critical.
14. My child is a pessimist.
15. My child fears the unexpected.
16. My child fears taking reasonable risks.
17. My child is not a self-sufficient person.
18. My child is not assertive.
19. My child cannot stand being alone.
20. My child fears being independent.
21. My child is an approval-seeking person.
22. My child gets in "over her head" and becomes overcommitted.
23. My child is a perfectionist and must have things just right.
24. My child is not a spiritual person.
25. My child does not respect or trust authority figures.
26. My child tends to engage in black-and-white thinking.
27. My child has a high activity level.
28. My child is an impatient person.
29. My child is easily frustrated.
30. My child favors immediate over delayed gratification.
31. My child is a compulsive person.
32. My child tends to "overdo it" or use things excessively .
33. My child is not determined, persistent, or motivated to achieve.

34. My child has difficulty finding pleasurable activities.
35. My child is not involved in school activities.
36. My child has little intellectual curiosity and little confidence academically.
37. My child dislikes school, has difficulty concentrating, and dislikes hard thinking.
38. My child has ineffective work and study habits.
39. My child is not organized and orderly.
40. My child engages in wishful thinking and seeks magical solutions to any problem.
41. My child is adventurous and thrill-seeking, enjoys risk-taking.
42. My child is self-centered.
43. My child is not a good listener and appears to know it all.
44. My child does not ask for or accept help.
45. My child appears aloof and indifferent.
46. My child has a lack of empathy for the feelings of others.
47. My child is tough and hard, rather than considerate and tender.
48. My child does not show gratitude.
49. My child has no sense of humor.
50. My child is excitable, high-strung, and easily angered.
51. My child does not express his true feelings and thoughts.
52. My child often lies and cheats.
53. My child is dishonest with others.
54. My child harbors resentments.
55. My child does not have any close friends.
56. My child is concerned with her image.
57. My child is demanding of others.
58. My child is irresponsible.
59. My child has had a difficult temperament since early in life.
60. My child tends to be a resistive and reactive person.

61. My child is disobedient and rebellious.
62. My child wants to do things her way and is unconventional.
63. My child gets easily frustrated over seemingly small matters .
64. My child blames others for his circumstances or situations.
65. My child spends time on the "pity pot" and feels sorry for herself.
66. My child puts things out of his mind and denies they exist.
67. My child has a hard time accepting responsibility.
68. My child thinks his fate is controlled by external circumstances rather than himself.
69. My child is insensitive to punishment.
70. My child feels anxious.
71. My child feels angry.
72. My child feels victimized.
73. My child feels stressed.
74. My child feels tense.
75. My child feels bored.
76. My child feels emotionally numb.
77. My child feels depressed.
78. My child feels empty.
79. My child feels inadequate.
80. My child feels trapped—like there's "no way out."
81. My child feels overwhelmed.
82. My child feels powerless.
83. My child feels her life has no purpose.
84. My child feels his life has little meaning.
85. My child feels shame.
86. My child feels too dependent.
87. My child feels isolated.

88. My child feels lonely.
89. My child feels rejected.
90. My child feels hopeless.
91. My child feels helpless.
92. My child feels like a failure.
93. My child feels unvalued and unaccepted.
94. My child is noncompliant and difficult to control.
95. My child is fearful, anxious, and sensitive.
96. My child has temper tantrums.
97. My child is strong-willed.
98. My child is having more trouble than her schoolmates learning to read and spell.

Home Environment At-Risk Characteristics

Children with parents, grandparents, foster parents, or siblings displaying antisocial behavior are at greater risk of developing AOD problems than other young people. There is also evidence that families with poor parenting skills have a disproportionately higher risk of having children who use AOD.

99. Your child was neither planned nor wanted by her mother.
100. Your child's mother suffered from AOD abuse, depression, or other problem that interfered with the care of your child.
101. Your child's parents had high expectations for his performance.
102. The parental discipline of your child was overly strict or lax.
103. Your child spends the majority of time unsupervised.
104. Your child was not nurtured or taught personal values or life skills by her parents.
105. The family's communications included put-downs and conflicts.
106. Your child's parents/caretakers lacked parenting skills to skillfully handle noncompliance in your child.
107. Your child was physically or verbally abused.
108. Your child was sexually abused.
109. Your child's parents openly used alcohol, illegal drugs, or prescription mind-altering drugs in front of him.
110. Your child's parents gave or allowed her to use alcohol or mind-altering drugs.
111. Your child does not share his thoughts and feelings with at least one family member.
112. You do not let your child know in advance what kind of behavior you expect.
113. You don't usually keep track of where your child is, what she is doing, and whom her friends are.
114. You do not praise your child for doing well.
115. When your child breaks family rules, you are not consistent and controlled in your punishment.

School At-Risk Characteristics

In the earliest school grades, even kindergarten, children at risk may be distinguished from others by their aggressiveness, antisocial behavior, combination of shyness and aggression, and problems adjusting to school. These children may have already been identified by school authorities as being at risk for later difficulties. If your child has any of these characteristics and you identify them, you will be able to help him change the attitude and behaviors that might otherwise lead to AOD abuse.

116. Your child dislikes school.
117. Your child has few friends at school.
118. Your child is not active in extracurricular activities.
119. Your child has poor academic achievement.
120. Your child is often willfully absent from school.
121. Your child is in a resource classroom for behaviorally disordered children.
122. The classrooms are overcrowded (35 or more children per teacher).
123. Teacher and school morale are low.
124. Your child misbehaves in school.
125. Alcohol and drugs are readily available at school.
126. Rules concerning delinquent behavior and school misbehavior are not consistently enforced.

Peer At-Risk Characteristics

One significant at-risk characteristic is the AOD-related attitude and behaviors of your child's best friends. Another is her preference of being with peers, choosing to get close to them instead of adults. Children whose best friends use AOD and those who choose peers over adults are at increased risk of AOD use. Lastly, children with older siblings who use AOD are also more likely to become involved with AOD.

127. Your child's friends smoke tobacco.
128. Your child's friends smoke marijuana.
129. Your child's friends use alcohol.
130. Your child's friends use a variety of illegal drugs.
131. Your child's friends believe it is okay to smoke tobacco and use alcohol and illegal drugs.
132. Your child's friends are thrillseekers in destructive or dangerous ways.
133. Your child's friends are independent and rebellious youth.
134. Your child's friends are often in trouble with the law.

Community At-Risk Characteristics

Community characteristics are often associated with delinquency and the development of child AOD abuse. For example, poverty and deprivation appear to be strongly associated with persistent AOD abuse and delinquent activity. Also, communities with significant residential mobility frequently show higher rates of crime, delinquency, and AOD abuse. Ironically, mobility may also reduce drug use by moving children away from their AOD-using peers. While social disorganization and deprivation increase the risk of AOD problems, high levels of AOD problems cause social disorganization. In either case, the coping abilities and opportunities necessary for success are diminished.

135. Your child lives in a community that condones or accepts heavy alcohol use.
136. Your child lives in a community that is passive or accepts the use of illegal drugs or prescription drugs without a doctor's consent.
137. Your child lives in a community that is disorganized and disrupted.
138. The community has few recreational, social, or cultural activities for your child.
139. Your child has had little opportunity to get involved in community activities because of frequent moves.
140. Your community has little economic opportunity for young people.

You have now completed the ARI and identified your child's at-risk characteristics. Your next task is to convert the characteristics into prevention objectives.

Identification and Selection of Prevention Objectives for Your Child

By completing the ARI, you have classified an abundance of information about your child. The next step is convert the at-risk characteristics you have identified into prevention objectives. The process outlined below will show you how to do this with each of the 140 items. If you want to use this book again or share it with others, copy each of the four worksheets identified in the process.

Instructions

1. Identify your *true* and *often true* responses from the seven categories and list them on the worksheet on page 36.
2. Identify your *false* responses from the seven categories and list them on the worksheet on page 37.
3. Identify your *seldom true* and *don't know* responses from the seven categories and list them on the worksheet on page 38.
4. Review your *true* and *often true* responses.

   These responses represent negative at-risk characteristics that can be *converted* into practical prevention objectives. For example, if you have responded *true* and *often true* to item #94, "My child is noncompliant and difficult to control," simply identify and write out the response to that characteristic. The prevention objective, in this case, might be to work with your child to help her become more responsive and compliant to expectations. If you have responded *true* and *often true* to item #42, "My child is self-centered," the objective involves helping your child develop a more sharing and caring attitude toward others. If you have responded *true* and *often true* to item #119, "My child has poor academic achievement," the objective would be to get more involved with your child's academic potential and school work. Place the characteristics you have identified with your *true* and *often true* responses on the "Objectives to Prevent Your Child's AOD Abuse" worksheet on page 39.
5. Review your *false* responses. These responses represent positive characteristics that can also be converted into prevention objectives. For example, if you have responded *false* to item #42, "My child is self-centered," change the item into the prevention objective, "My child is not self-centered." Continue to support this attitude about your child. If you have responded *false* to item #53, "My child is dishonest with others," convert the objective to, "My child is honest," and continue to reinforce this attitude. If you have responded *false* to item #138, "The community has few recreational, social, or cultural activities for your child," convert the objective to, "Get my child involved in appro-

priate activities." Place the characteristics you have identified as your *false* responses on the section, "Objectives to Prevent Your Child's AOD Abuse" worksheet on page 39.

6. Your responses in Category 1 and Category 2 are based on historical issues that cannot be changed. They may, however, be converted into objectives by talking with your child about the potential at-risk characteristic of each response.
7. Review your list of *seldom true* and *don't know* responses. You will need to monitor and give more thought to these characteristics before determining whether or not to use them as prevention objectives. After you have decided, select the responses that could be appropriately converted into prevention objectives.
8. Using the "Objectives To Prevent Your Child's AOD Abuse" worksheet, arrange the prevention objectives by priority. Identify a starting objective and determine the sequence of the others. Sort out daily, weekly, or monthly objectives. Determine how you will achieve each objective. Consider the following examples:
    - Talking with your child about the at-risk characteristic(s) in a sharing, caring, and objective manner.
    - Gathering further information about child-rearing effectiveness and child or teen AOD abuse. Certainly, you have made a good start by reading this book. Don't forget to check the recommended readings and bibliography for additional material.
    - Getting involved with school and community organizations that work with your child. Take an active role.
    - Attending workshops at the school and within the community, such as STEP, *Systematic Training for Effective Parenting*. Identify an implementation date for each objective. Monitor and evaluate your progress for each objective.
9. If your prevention efforts are successful, consider Strategy 2 for additional information. It has a number of possible prevention objectives that you may decide to use on your master sheet.
10. Use the evaluation instrument on a periodic basis. If you detect AOD abuse and a consultation with a professional is recommended, use Strategy 3.

List Your *True* and *Often True* Responses

1. ______________________________
2. ______________________________
3. ______________________________
4. ______________________________
5. ______________________________
6. ______________________________
7. ______________________________
8. ______________________________
9. ______________________________
10. ______________________________
11. ______________________________
12. ______________________________
13. ______________________________
14. ______________________________
15. ______________________________
16. ______________________________
17. ______________________________
18. ______________________________
19. ______________________________
20. ______________________________
21. ______________________________
22. ______________________________
23. ______________________________
24. ______________________________
25. ______________________________

List Your *False* Responses

1. ______________________________
2. ______________________________
3. ______________________________
4. ______________________________
5. ______________________________
6. ______________________________
7. ______________________________
8. ______________________________
9. ______________________________
10. ______________________________
11. ______________________________
12. ______________________________
13. ______________________________
14. ______________________________
15. ______________________________
16. ______________________________
17. ______________________________
18. ______________________________
19. ______________________________
20. ______________________________
21. ______________________________
22. ______________________________
23. ______________________________
24. ______________________________
25. ______________________________

List Your *Seldom True* and *Don't Know* Responses

1. ______
2. ______
3. ______
4. ______
5. ______
6. ______
7. ______
8. ______
9. ______
10. ______
11. ______
12. ______
13. ______
14. ______
15. ______
16. ______
17. ______
18. ______
19. ______
20. ______
21. ______
22. ______
23. ______
24. ______
25. ______

Objectives to Prevent Your Child's AOD Abuse

OBJECTIVE	PRIORITY	BY WHEN
Work with Mary to help her become more responsive and compliant to expectations.	2	Oct. 12
Help Mary develop a more sharing and caring attitude about others.	3	Nov. 7
Get more involved with Mary's academic potential and school work.	1	Sept. 15

The At-Risk Inventory Answer Sheet

1. F T ?
2. F T ?
3. F T ?
4. F T ?
5. F T ?
6. F T ?
7. F T ?
8. F T ?
9. F T ?
10. F T ST OT ?
11. F T ST OT ?
12. F T ST OT ?
13. F T ST OT ?
14. F T ST OT ?
15. F T ST OT ?
16. F T ST OT ?
17. F T ST OT ?
18. F T ST OT ?
19. F T ST OT ?
20. F T ST OT ?
21. F T ST OT ?
22. F T ST OT ?
23. F T ST OT ?
24. F T ?
25. F T ST OT ?
26. F T ST OT ?
27. F T ST OT ?
28. F T ST OT ?
29. F T ST OT ?
30. F T ST OT ?
31. F T ST OT ?
32. F T ST OT ?
33. F T ST OT ?
34. F T ST OT ?
35. F T ST OT ?
36. F T ST OT ?
37. F T ST OT ?
38. F T ST OT ?
39. F T ST OT ?
40. F T ST OT ?
41. F T ST OT ?
42. F T ST OT ?
43. F T ST OT ?
44. F T ST OT ?
45. F T ST OT ?
46. F T ST OT ?
47. F T ST OT ?
48. F T ST OT ?
49. F T ST OT ?
50. F T ST OT ?
51. F T ST OT ?
52. F T ST OT ?
53. F T ST OT ?
54. F T ST OT ?
55. F T ST OT ?
56. F T ST OT ?
57. F T ST OT ?
58. F T ST OT ?
59. F T ST OT ?
60. F T ST OT ?
61. F T ST OT ?
62. F T ST OT ?
63. F T ST OT ?
64. F T ST OT ?
65. F T ST OT ?
66. F T ST OT ?
67. F T ST OT ?
68. F T ST OT ?
69. F T ST OT ?
70. F T ST OT ?
71. F T ST OT ?
72. F T ST OT ?
73. F T ST OT ?
74. F T ST OT ?
75. F T ST OT ?
76. F T ST OT ?
77. F T ST OT ?
78. F T ST OT ?
79. F T ST OT ?
80. F T ST OT ?
81. F T ST OT ?
82. F T ST OT ?
83. F T ST OT ?
84. F T ST OT ?
85. F T ST OT ?
86. F T ST OT ?
87. F T ST OT ?
88. F T ST OT ?
89. F T ST OT ?
90. F T ST OT ?
91. F T ST OT ?
92. F T ST OT ?
93. F T ST OT ?
94. F T ST OT ?
95. F T ST OT ?
96. F T ST OT ?
97. F T ST OT ?
98. F T ?
99. F T ?
100. F T ?
101. F T ?
102. F T ST OT ?
103. F T ST OT ?
104. F T ?
105. F T ST OT ?
106. F T ?
107. F T ST OT ?
108. F T ?
109. F T ST OT ?
110. F T ST OT ?
111. F T ST OT ?
112. F T ST OT ?
113. F T ST OT ?
114. F T ST OT ?
115. F T ST OT ?
116. F T ST OT ?
117. F T ?
118. F T ST OT ?
119. F T ST OT ?
120. F T ST OT ?
121. F T ?
122. F T ?
123. F T ?
124. F T ST OT ?
125. F T ST OT ?
126. F T ?
127. F T ST OT ?
128. F T ST OT ?
129. F T ST OT ?
130. F T ST OT ?
131. F T ?
132. F T ST OT ?
133. F T ST OT ?
134. F T ST OT ?
135. F T ?
136. F T ?
137. F T ?
138. F T ?
139. F T ?
140. F T ?

Strategy 2

Designing a Personalized Plan to Prevent Your Child's AOD Abuse

Unfortunately, there is no strategy that will ensure 100% effectiveness for the prevention of child alcohol and other drug (AOD) abuse. One thing is certain, however: The "horrors of addiction" do not work. Research has shown that young people cannot be scared into abstinence. In addition, school efforts have had some general impact in preventing AOD use, but how much or how little is debatable. Without a doubt, the most effective way to prevent child or teen AOD abuse is through education and training of parents and caregivers. With information and a plan of action, you can have the greatest positive impact in reducing the destructive consequences of AOD abuse among young people, starting with your own child.

This strategy is the starting point. With this strategy, you will learn how to design and use your own personalized plan to maximize your efforts in preventing your child's AOD abuse. Your plan will be based on tasks and activities you select from the comprehensive 115-item Prevention Inventory.

First, though, you will learn why young people use AOD and why your child is vulnerable. This discussion will give you an idea of the dynamics, pressures, and persuasion involved in your child's decisions about AOD use. Next, you will learn how and where AOD are available to your child, which will help you in your prevention efforts. This will be followed by a discussion about the types of your responses or nonresponses that may increase the likelihood of child or teen AOD abuse. Then you will complete the inventory to select the tasks and activities that are suitable for your child.

Once you have completed the Prevention Inventory, you will list your responses on three separate worksheets. Next, you will learn how to convert your responses into personalized prevention objectives. Finally, you will place your objectives on a master sheet and assign a priority value and completion date for each one. At the end of the process, you will have up to 115 personalized objectives that you can use to prevent your child's AOD abuse.

If the strategy is successful, you will be encouraged to consider Strategy 1 for additional information. It has a number of excellent tasks and activities that you may decide to use on your master sheet. Use the evaluation instrument on a periodic basis. If you detect AOD abuse and a consultation with a professional is recommended, use Strategy 3.

Why Children Use AOD

Children cite many reasons for using AOD. According to research, the major reason why children use AOD is because they are curious about the effects and have a natural tendency to experiment. Actually, curiosity and wonderment are the first basic steps to wisdom and success in life. Ironically, we want children to be curious about things like reading, writing, and arithmetic—but not about AOD. This is not a realistic expectation, however. For most young people, what feels good must be good, and few think they will ever die from that feeling. In this case, curiosity and experimentation, coupled with feelings of immortality, can prove to be dangerous.

Peer group acceptance is also high on the list of reasons. We all need to feel a sense of belonging, not only to our families but also to our peer group. We strive to be regarded as worthwhile by our friends. Children and teens are no different. In fact, they feel that pressure more strongly than do adults. Although many will deny it, friends can have a dramatic influence on children's decisions about AOD use.

Adults also influence children's decisions, and many children who pattern habits learned from adults use this as an excuse or "cop out." But this thinking contains an element of truth. How and why adults use AOD, coupled with the commercialism and marketing of these products, do indeed help mold a child's point of view. Lastly, young people use AOD to feel the excitement of risks, to feel important and be good at something, to relieve boredom, to feel less inhibited, and to escape family pressure.

These reasons pertain to underlying psychological motivations and needs. After experimenting with AOD, children begin to learn many things. They can be successful, pretty, handsome and popular, or avoid and escape unpleasant, painful problems by using AOD. This attitude can have dangerous consequences.

Although this information may make you want to change your child's healthy curiosity about life, you should not do so. But you can help your child make positive decisions about AOD use and good choices about friends. You can also set an example as an adult and teach him how to effectively deal with life's problems. To begin, though, you need to be aware of his vulnerabilities.

Why Your Child Is Vulnerable to AOD Abuse

Childhood and adolescence are periods of dramatic emotional, social, and physical growth. While developing from a tentative, dependent position into the role of an independent adult, today's young person lives in an increasingly complicated world and complex society where seemingly the only thing *constant* is *change,* a concept borrowed from Alvin Toffler in his prophetic best-selling book, *Future Shock.* He states

> What joins all these.... (i.e. daily events) is the *roaring current of change* so powerful today that it overturns institutions, shifts our values and shrivels our roots. Change is the process by which the future invades our lives, and it is important to look at it closely, not merely from the grand perspectives of history, but also from the vantage point of the living, breathing individuals who experience it. The acceleration of change in our time is, itself, an elemental force. This accelerative thrust has personal and psychological, as well as sociological consequences. [Toffler 1970, pp. 1-2]

The American family structure reflects one dramatic example of the "roaring current of change." Over the last 30 years, the family has become more mobile and transient, the divorce rate has skyrocketed, and the roles of men and women have significantly changed. Because of these changes, children are less supervised than in preceding generations. There is also less communication about family values and AOD issues, as revealed in the ABC News/*Washington Post* poll* released in 1996. According to the poll, the following data reveal this trend:

- Sixty-two percent of parents say their teenagers feel comfortable talking with them about drugs, but only 45% of teens say the same.
- Most parents say they've had a serious talk with their children about illegal drugs, but a majority of teens say that's not so.
- Exactly 85% of parents *say* they have had a serious talk with their child about drugs, but children may not have heard it that way. Only 45% of the teenagers in the poll recalled a serious talk.
- Most teens who did talk with their parents about drugs say it helped, and half say it helped a lot.

With less supervision and communication happening during an often difficult time of childhood development and growth, a young person is exposed and vulnerable to numerous forms of pressure and persuasion influencing her choices about AOD. For example, the young person experiences an unprecedented cli-

---

* American parents and their children have different perceptions about various aspects of America's drug problem and how parents respond. This survey, conducted by *The Washington Post* and ABC News, polled 618 parents of teenagers and 527 young people (ages 12 to 17), including 441 teenage children of the parents surveyed [Morin & Brossard 1997, p. A1].

mate of intensive peer group pressure. Even if a family is close and stable, the child is still exposed to the daily interaction and influence of her friends.

Television also represents a significant source of pressure and persuasion:

- The average child sees more than 20,000 commercials each year. By age 21, the average viewer will have seen 1 million television commercials.
- Children see at least one hour of commercials for every five hours of programs they watch on commercial TV.
- Teens see 100,000 alcohol commercials before they reach drinking age [Electronic Policy Network, no date].*

This includes beer and wine advertisements and over-the-counter drugs. A number of commercials, using hidden persuasion techniques, depict handsome, beautiful, and athletic people drinking alcohol in various social situations. Other commercials reflect the attitude that a chemical solution or pill exists for almost any ailment known to mankind. Advertisements and commercials beg viewers to believe that if you don't feel well, take a drug and you will. Further appeals and messages are offered to children in the lyrics of rap, hard or acid rock music, and at live rock concerts held throughout the country.

Finally, children are exposed to traumatic, dramatic international, national, and local events on an immediate, daily basis via mass media coverage. Unfortunately, these appeals and messages often go unheeded and undisputed by parents and other caregivers of children. During a difficult period of growth and development in a constantly changing environment, littered with and bombarded by commercial appeals, daily peer pressure, exposure to dramatic events, rock music and hidden persuasion, your child can be greatly influenced to try AOD.

How and Where Alcohol-Drugs Are Available to Your Child

Do you know where children get alcohol and other drugs? You may be surprised. Listed below are the sources of AOD:

- **Friend's house.** A primary source for alcohol, regardless of the friend's age.
- **Parties.** Buying a ticket or pitching in to buy pills, pot, or alcohol at parties in homes or rented facilities.
- **Home.** The refrigerator, the liquor cabinet, at cocktail parties, from older brothers and sisters, or the medicine cabinet.

---

* For more information, contact the Center for Media Education, a national nonprofit organization dedicated to improving the quality of electronic media, especially on behalf of children and families, at 2120 L Street NW, Suite 200, Washington, DC 20037, 202/331-7833, fax: 202/331-7841.

- **School.** From child or teen "pushers," others sharing AOD stolen from home, and young adults old enough to buy alcohol legally.
- **Liquor stores.** Using false identification, asking adults to buy the liquor, or stealing from unsuspecting adults.
- **Shoplifting.** Stealing alcohol and nonprescription drugs from supermarkets or drug stores or shoplifting items that may be converted into cash to buy or trade for AOD.
- **Baby-sitting.** Drinking or using drugs in the employer's home or stealing from the liquor supply or medicine cabinet to use or "push" at a later date.

Typical Responses to Avoid

Apathy, denial, impatience, and guilt are four typical responses—and doomsday pitfalls to avoid. The responses are defined and described below.

- **Apathy.** The qualities of a solid family structure and stable middle class environment do not necessarily protect against child AOD abuse. Although surveys and statistics show that child AOD is an "equal opportunity employer," many parents and other caregivers act unrealistically complacent about the potential or existence of AOD use by their children.
- **Denial.** Often adults regard child drinking as a stage or accept AOD-related behaviors as normal. Remember, though, that today's young person is exposed to unprecedented pressure, persuasion, and change in a world where AOD are immediately available and accessible. Do not deny the possibility of your child's AOD abuse. Presuming that AOD-related behaviors are simply your child's way of "sowing oats" is naïve and dangerous.
- **Guilt.** Adults tend to assume guilt for the child's choice to use AOD. They wonder, "Where did we go wrong?" Unfortunately, this notion is reinforced in many of the pop psychology books sold throughout the country. Instead of trying to analyze what went wrong, remember that you are a loving, caring, and responsible adult concerned about the well-being and healthy growth of your child. Get off of the unjustifiable guilt trip, obtain relevant information, and do something constructive about your child's choice to abuse AOD.
- **Impatience.** Adults must take the time and make the effort to do what is necessary to prevent child or teen AOD abuse. Regardless of what you may have read or heard, there are no easy, overnight solutions. It will take time to investigate and evaluate your present needs and circumstances. You will also need to learn about the tasks, activities, and strategies in preventing AOD abuse by your child. Your success will depend upon your commitment.

The Prevention Inventory

Instructions

The following inventory consists of 115 questions that will help you design a prevention plan. Respond to the questions with Y = Yes, N = No, or ? to indicate that you don't know. As you will see later, each question can be converted into a prevention objective that you can incorporate into your own prevention plan. Because you may want to use this book again or share it with others, copy and use the Prevention Inventory Answer Sheet on page 59.

If you are going to have children:

1. Will you have regular prenatal care during your pregnancy?
2. Will you avoid all alcohol during your pregnancy?
3. Will you avoid smoking or using any form of speed (tobacco, diet pills, cocaine, amphetamines) during your pregnancy?
4. Will you eat and sleep well and stay healthy during the pregnancy?

Have you taken your own personal inventory concerning:

5. The extent of your parenting knowledge, attitudes, and skills?
6. Your personal parenting characteristics?
7. How you feel about your child's characteristics?
8. How you respond to stress?
9. Whether or not you are supportive of your child?
10. Your work characteristics?
11. Your household characteristics?
12. Your marital characteristics?
13. Your cultural and religious values?

Do you know:

14. The extent of child AOD abuse?
15. The meaning of an addiction and the addiction process?
16. Why people get addicted?

17. How to determine if your child is at risk for AOD abuse?
18. How to maximize your efforts in preventing your child's AOD abuse?
19. Why your child is vulnerable to AOD abuse?
20. How and where AOD are available to your child?
21. Why children use AOD?
22. How to detect AOD abuse in your home?
23. The signs of other children's AOD abuse?
24. How to determine if your child abuses AOD?
25. How to consult with a professional to determine if your child has an AOD problem?
26. How and when to select a counselor?
27. What to expect from counseling?
28. How to confront your child if he abuses AOD?
29. How to make a contract offering consequences for abusing AOD?
30. How, when, and why to use an intervention with your child if she is abusing AOD *and* how and where to refer her for treatment?
31. The criteria for an effective inpatient/residential treatment program?
32. What to expect before, during, and after inpatient/residential treatment?
33. Which drugs do what?
34. Terms related to child or teen AOD use and abuse?

Does your child:

35. Have family members who are supportive and caring?
36. Have extended family members or family friends with whom he is close?
37. Like his parents?
38. Receive regular praise for progress in his development and education?
39. Have a confidant in the home?
40. Have clear roles and responsibilities in the home?

Have you helped your child develop the ability:

41. To adapt her attitude and behavior to new or changing circumstances?
42. To effectively deal with and resist the frequently subtle media appeals to use AOD?
43. To develop skills needed to resist peer appeals to use AOD?
44. To use healthy ways to process anger in situations that arouse anger?
45. To share wants, needs, ideas, and feelings in an honest, accurate, and responsible manner without denying her own right to express herself or the rights of others to be respected?
46. To give and receive information, signals, or messages by talking, writing or gesturing?
47. To respond to and contend with stress-related situations in a healthy and constructive manner?
48. To develop and use contingency plan(s) in a stress-related situation if the original plan or plans fail?
49. To develop and use a format intended to remind or warn her of potential conflicts or problems?
50. To organize and plan long-term, intermediate, and immediate goals and objectives?
51. To use investigative, analytical, and evaluative techniques to resolve conflicts and problems?
52. To regulate and accept responsibility for his behavior?
53. To constructively interact with people as well as to adapt and conform to the common needs and standards of society?
54. To identify and use specific techniques or strategies to reduce or eliminate stress?
55. To identify and use decisionmaking skills?

Have you encouraged your child to develop:

56. Good verbal skills?
57. A flexible thinking pattern?
58. Pride in his appearance?
59. Good social skills?
60. A motivation to succeed?
61. A healthy lifestyle?
62. A positive attitude about learning and responding to his teachers?

Have you told your child that:

63. Drinking alcohol or using other drugs can be abusive, because it can bring harm to the user or other people?
64. Any drinking is abuse, because it can affect growth and development?
65. Any drinking is inappropriate, because it is illegal if she is under 21?
66. Any drinking or other drug use is improper, because it can harm an unborn baby?
67. People with a family history of alcoholism may be prone to abuse?
68. Engaging in sports while under the influence of AOD is dangerous?
69. Driving or operating machinery while drinking or using drugs is dangerous?
70. Any drinking or other drug use can be abuse?

General Questions:

71. Do you limit yourself to occasional social drinking with no more than one or two drinks, no more than once or twice a week?
72. Do you talk to your child about abstaining from smoking and refrain from doing so yourself?
73. Are family meetings scheduled regularly to discuss and make decisions about issues that involve the entire family?
74. Does your family have regular daily routines and family rituals that are rarely disrupted?
75. Do family meetings provide opportunities for your child to become involved in decisionmaking?
76. Is your family's communication style characterized by politeness, support, and caring for the other members?
77. Do you explore alternatives by brainstorming with your child to encourage creative thinking?
78. Do you teach decisionmaking by involving your child in decisionmaking processes?
79. Do you help your child choose a solution to his problems?
80. Do you help your child examine the possible consequences of his choices and decisions?
81. Does your family expect no use of any illegal drugs by anyone and no use of alcohol by anyone under the legal drinking age?
82. Does your family have a clear stand against AOD use reinforced by clear and enforceable consequences?
83. Does your child know what the consequences of using AOD will be before the misbehavior occurs?
84. Do you teach decisionmaking as early as possible by allowing your child to make choices consistent with his age and level of maturity?
85. Do you use democratic and skillful discipline techniques with your child?
86. Do you listen to your child to understand him and help him clarify his feelings?
87. Do you have an understanding of your child's positive and negative feelings and the circumstances that cause them?

88. Do you talk with your child about advertisements and commercials to strengthen her ability to resist hidden persuasive appeals?
89. Have you educated your child about illegal choices and their consequences?
90. Have you educated your child about sex and appropriate sexual behaviors consistent with his age?
91. Have you educated your child about AOD in a manner appropriate for her age?
92. Do you help your child process television programs to sort out the difference between reality and fiction?
93. Are the majority of your child's friends good kids who do well academically and have no problems with the law?
94. Do the majority of your child's friends believe it is wrong to use tobacco, alcohol, or drugs?
95. Do the majority of your child's friends not use tobacco, alcohol, or drugs?
96. Do you provide your child with accurate statistical information about the extent of use by his peers?
97. Do you help your child focus on and engage in healthy activities, including AOD-free parties, as alternatives to unhealthy ones?
98. Do you monitor your child's whereabouts to give her the opportunity to demonstrate the ability to handle increasing amounts of freedom?
99. Do you monitor your child's whereabouts to be reasonably assured of his safety?
100. Does your child like school?
101. Is your child motivated to do well in school?
102. Is your child active in extracurricular activities?
103. Does your child currently have adults at school who have taken a special interest in her and her talents?
104. Do you assist your child in academic areas where he is having problems and help him with homework?
105. Does your child's school have a clear policy of AOD nonuse at school and an effective discipline policy?
106. Does your child's school have an effective course of AOD education consisting of ten or more sessions per year?

107. Does your child have a number of peer groups in the community with whom he is involved?
108. Is your child involved in a number of community clubs and activities?
109. Does your community have a clear message that AOD abuse is unhealthy and unwise?
110. Is access to alcohol and illegal drugs restricted for both young people and adults in your community?
111. Is your family active in civic, social, cultural, educational, or service groups in the community?
112. Are you and your child actively involved in a church or religious organization?
113. Do you read books and other publications about child or teen AOD abuse?
114. Do you have an understanding of current AOD messages and slang terms?
115. Do you attend workshops or seminars on the topic of child or teen AOD abuse?

Designing Your Personalized Prevention Plan

By completing the inventory, you have classified an abundance of information about your child. Now you must convert your answers into objectives and design a plan to prevent your child's AOD abuse. The process outlined below will show you how to do this with each of the 115 items. If you want to use this book again or share it with others, copy each of the four worksheets involved in the process.

Instructions

1. Identify your *no* responses and list them on the worksheet on page 55.
2. Identify your *yes* responses and list them on the worksheet on page 56.
3. Identify your *don't know* responses and list them on the worksheet on page 57.
4. Review the questions you responded to with *no*. Each of your *no* responses can be *converted* into prevention objectives by using counterpoints of the statement. For example, if you responded *no* to question #100 that your child does not like school, the prevention objective involves working with your child to help her become more responsive to the school environment.

   If you responded *no* to question #79 about helping your child choose solutions for problems, the prevention objective involves becoming more involved with your child in his decisionmaking and problemsolving situations. If you responded *no* to question #40 about your child having clear roles and responsibilities in the home, the prevention objective involves clarifying his role in the family and identifying specific tasks for him to complete.

   Now select the questions that could be *appropriately* converted into prevention objectives for your child. Then place the objectives on the "Personalized Prevention Plan for Your Child" on page 58.
5. Review the questions you have identified with your *yes* responses. These responses represent positive questions that can also be converted into prevention objectives. For example, if you responded *yes* to question #59 about encouraging your child to develop good social skills, change the question into the prevention objective. Affirm your belief in your child's social skills and support your child on this attitude.

   If you responded *yes* to question #105 about your child's school AOD policy discipline procedures, change the question into a prevention objective. Support the school's AOD policy. If you responded *yes* to question #80 about helping your child examine the likely consequences of his choices and decisions, turn it into a prevention objective. Help your child examine the likely consequences of his choices and decisions. Next place the objectives on the "Personalized Prevention Plan for Your Child" on page 58.

6. Review your list of *don't know* responses. You will need to give more thought to these questions before determining whether or not to use them as prevention objectives. After you have decided, select the responses that could be *appropriately* converted into prevention objectives. Place each objective in your *yes* or *no* response list.

   The objectives you have identified with your *yes* responses are those you will use in your prevention plan. Also, select the responses from your *no* list that could be *appropriately* converted into prevention objectives for your child in your home setting and place those prevention objectives in the "Personalized Prevention Plan for Your Child" on page 58.

7. Use the "Personalized Prevention Plan for Your Child" worksheet to complete the following steps:
   - Arrange the prevention objectives on a priority basis. Identify which objective you will start with and determine the sequence of the others.
   - Sort out daily, weekly, or monthly objectives.
   - Determine how you will achieve each objective. Consider using the following examples:

     Talk with your child about the at-risk characteristics in a caring and objective manner.

     Gather further information about parenting effectiveness and child or teen AOD abuse. Certainly, you have made a good start by reading this book. Don't forget to check out the recommended readings and bibliography in the back of this book.

     Get involved with school and community organizations that work with your child. Take an active role in your child's life. Attend workshops at the school and within the community such as *Systematic Training for Effective Parenting* (STEP).
   - Identify the implementation date for each objective.
   - Monitor and evaluate your progress for each objective.

8. If your prevention efforts are successful, consider Strategy 1 for additional information. It has a number of excellent tasks and activities that you may decide to use on your master sheet.

9. Use the evaluation instrument on a periodic basis. If you detect AOD abuse and a consultation with a professional is recommended, use Strategy 3.

List Your *No* Responses

1. ______
2. ______
3. ______
4. ______
5. ______
6. ______
7. ______
8. ______
9. ______
10. ______
11. ______
12. ______
13. ______
14. ______
15. ______
16. ______
17. ______
18. ______
19. ______
20. ______
21. ______
22. ______
23. ______
24. ______
25. ______

List Your *Yes* Responses

1. ____________________
2. ____________________
3. ____________________
4. ____________________
5. ____________________
6. ____________________
7. ____________________
8. ____________________
9. ____________________
10. ____________________
11. ____________________
12. ____________________
13. ____________________
14. ____________________
15. ____________________
16. ____________________
17. ____________________
18. ____________________
19. ____________________
20. ____________________
21. ____________________
22. ____________________
23. ____________________
24. ____________________
25. ____________________

List Your *Don't Know* Responses

1. ______________________________
2. ______________________________
3. ______________________________
4. ______________________________
5. ______________________________
6. ______________________________
7. ______________________________
8. ______________________________
9. ______________________________
10. ______________________________
11. ______________________________
12. ______________________________
13. ______________________________
14. ______________________________
15. ______________________________
16. ______________________________
17. ______________________________
18. ______________________________
19. ______________________________
20. ______________________________
21. ______________________________
22. ______________________________
23. ______________________________
24. ______________________________
25. ______________________________

Personalized Prevention Plan for Your Child

OBJECTIVE	PRIORITY	BY WHEN
Affirm my belief in John's social skills and support him on this attitude.	1	Feb. 2
Support the school's AOD policy.	3	Mar. 17
Help John examine the likely consequences of his choices and decisions.	2	Mar. 3

The Prevention Inventory Answer Sheet

1.	Y	N	?	32.	Y	N	?	63.	Y	N	?	94.	Y	N	?
2.	Y	N	?	33.	Y	N	?	64.	Y	N	?	95.	Y	N	?
3.	Y	N	?	34.	Y	N	?	65.	Y	N	?	96.	Y	N	?
4.	Y	N	?	35.	Y	N	?	66.	Y	N	?	97.	Y	N	?
5.	Y	N	?	36.	Y	N	?	67.	Y	N	?	98.	Y	N	?
6.	Y	N	?	37.	Y	N	?	68.	Y	N	?	99.	Y	N	?
7.	Y	N	?	38.	Y	N	?	69.	Y	N	?	100.	Y	N	?
8.	Y	N	?	39.	Y	N	?	70.	Y	N	?	101.	Y	N	?
9.	Y	N	?	40.	Y	N	?	71.	Y	N	?	102.	Y	N	?
10.	Y	N	?	41.	Y	N	?	72.	Y	N	?	103.	Y	N	?
11.	Y	N	?	42.	Y	N	?	73.	Y	N	?	104.	Y	N	?
12.	Y	N	?	43.	Y	N	?	74.	Y	N	?	105.	Y	N	?
13.	Y	N	?	44.	Y	N	?	75.	Y	N	?	106.	Y	N	?
14.	Y	N	?	45.	Y	N	?	76.	Y	N	?	107.	Y	N	?
15.	Y	N	?	46.	Y	N	?	77.	Y	N	?	108.	Y	N	?
16.	Y	N	?	47.	Y	N	?	78.	Y	N	?	109.	Y	N	?
17.	Y	N	?	48.	Y	N	?	79.	Y	N	?	110.	Y	N	?
18.	Y	N	?	49.	Y	N	?	80.	Y	N	?	111.	Y	N	?
19.	Y	N	?	50.	Y	N	?	81.	Y	N	?	112.	Y	N	?
20.	Y	N	?	51.	Y	N	?	82.	Y	N	?	113.	Y	N	?
21.	Y	N	?	52.	Y	N	?	83.	Y	N	?	114.	Y	N	?
22.	Y	N	?	53.	Y	N	?	84.	Y	N	?	115.	Y	N	?
23.	Y	N	?	54.	Y	N	?	85.	Y	N	?				
24.	Y	N	?	55.	Y	N	?	86.	Y	N	?				
25.	Y	N	?	56.	Y	N	?	87.	Y	N	?				
26.	Y	N	?	57.	Y	N	?	88.	Y	N	?				
27.	Y	N	?	58.	Y	N	?	89.	Y	N	?				
28.	Y	N	?	59.	Y	N	?	90.	Y	N	?				
29.	Y	N	?	60.	Y	N	?	91.	Y	N	?				
30.	Y	N	?	61.	Y	N	?	92.	Y	N	?				
31.	Y	N	?	62.	Y	N	?	93.	Y	N	?				

Strategy 3

Consulting with a Professional to Determine If Your Child Has an AOD Problem

Reading books like this one or attending workshops and support groups meetings, while excellent tasks and activities, do not make you an expert at dealing with your child's abuse of alcohol or other drugs (AOD). If you know your child is using AOD or is at high risk for abusing AOD, you should consult a mental health professional with expertise in child and teen AOD-related problems. The professional will help you sort out your feelings and observations so that you can determine what is best for your child. It will be one of the best investments you ever make.

Parents and caregivers are often reluctant to contact a professional about their child's AOD abuse for several reasons. They may be complacent about the consequences of their child's AOD use or regard it as a "rite of passage." They can also feel guilty about their child's choice to abuse AOD and be unwilling to seek professional help in fear of getting an angry response from their child or upsetting family accord. Additionally, financial limitations and the lack of direction can put professional assistance out of reach. The AOD problem does not go away and often gets much worse, however.

Using this strategy, you will be able to resolve any concerns you may have about seeking professional counseling. Specifically, you will learn how to select a professional for a consultation and how to make the best decision about your child's AOD abuse, regardless of the recommendations. You'll also learn what to expect from counseling and how you will be involved in the process. If counseling is not successful, you will have three other strategies to fall back on.

Selecting a Consultant

To select an appropriate and qualified mental health professional, obtain recommendations from the following:

- **A trusted friend who has experienced a similar situation**. Word of mouth from a close friend who has experienced a similar situation is not like money in the bank. But the reliability factor is better than most referral sources. You can get a firsthand, honest opinion based on actual experience. Just make sure the recommendation is for a consultant with expertise in child or teen AOD-related problems.

- **Your family physician**. Your doctor has daily contact with other medical and therapeutic professionals in the community and is often aware of who is the most effective. Get your doctor's opinion and add it to the list of your recommendations.
- **The mental health association in your community.** Contact your local mental health association. Share your concerns about your child's AOD situation and request a recommendation. A staff person is usually able to provide objective and impartial suggestions about a qualified mental health professional.
- **A community mental health center**. Your community or neighborhood area probably has a comprehensive mental health center. As nonprofit agencies, the centers help people with all types of problems, regardless of background and financial status. Call them and see if they have any recommendations or staff available to assist with your concerns.

Making Your Choice

You should now have a list of recommendations for qualified consultants. To select the one most appropriate for your needs, call each candidate and inquire about his/her qualifications and experience. There are several qualified professionals to consider: psychiatrists with medical degrees, psychologists with doctorate degrees, social workers, family and marriage counselors with a minimum of a master's degree, and other mental health therapists with a master's degree in an appropriate field. Regardless of the credentials, make sure that each prospect has expertise in child AOD abuse and is a licensed or certified professional in your state. If not, move on to the next candidate. Also, ask about the fee structure and the availability of the professional. After you have completed this process, you should have the essential information to make your choice. Once you have made your decision, call for an appointment.

Consulting with a Professional

At the consultation, be prepared to provide any relevant input about your child and his AOD use. Write down any observations in advance. Discuss what efforts you have made with your child to this point. Anything you have done may count, so be able to describe what you've done, how you've done it, and whether or not it worked.

If an AOD abuse problem exists with your child, the professional will probably recommend a certain type of program within a continuum of care. The continuum of care is the complete range of programs and services available in a mental health organization that offers a variety of treatment options, combining inpatient and outpatient care or providing day and night outpatient schedules. The options include:

- **Individual sessions at an office or outpatient clinic.** Sessions last usually under an hour with the number of visits per week dependent upon the needs of the child or teen.
- **An intensive outpatient program typically lasting six to eight weeks.** Clients attend several sessions a week during the afternoon or evening hours so that they can continue with school and meet other daily responsibilities.
- **Individualized case management services in a home-based treatment program.** Specially trained individuals coordinate counseling, financial, legal, and medical services in a treatment program to help the child or teen live successfully at home and in the community.
- **A day treatment program or partial hospitalization**. This intensive treatment program provides psychiatric care with case management services and special education. The child usually attends five days per week.
- **A therapeutic group home or community residence**. This therapeutic program usually includes eight to ten children or adolescents living in a home that is typically linked with a day treatment program or specialized educational program.
- **Hospital treatment.** The patients receive comprehensive psychiatric treatment in a hospital. The length of treatment ranges from a few days for acute care up to 30 days for intermediate care.
- **A crisis residence.** This setting provides short-term crisis intervention, acute stabilization, and detoxification services and treatment usually for fewer than 15 days. Patients receive 24-hour-per-day supervision.

8. **A residential treatment facility.** Seriously disturbed patients receive intensive and comprehensive psychiatric treatment in a campuslike setting on a long-term basis. Because most mental health organizations do not have every type of program in the continuum, you may be referred to appropriate community resources and services.

Making Your Decision about AOD Treatment

You can use the Recommendation Worksheet on page 65 as your research blueprint to help you make the best decision possible about treatment options. It provides the questions you should ask during the recommendation process. The format is easy to follow. First, the question to be asked is presented. Next, the reason for asking the question is explained. Then a brief space is given for the consultant's answers. Use a separate sheet to record the answers, which will guide you in making your decision.

Unless there is an immediate need to hospitalize your child, do not be pressured into a treatment decision. Instead, complete the separate answer sheet and review the information at home. Compare the consultant's answers with the reasons for asking the questions. You may want some extra time for a family discussion or additional reading and thinking before you make your decision. Then make your decision. If questions or doubts persist, however, get a second opinion. Do not accept any recommendation carte blanche. Be prepared to ask questions and clarify answers. As noted, there are several options for AOD abuse treatment and the decision to entrust your child to any type of treatment deserves your serious consideration.

The Recommendation Worksheet

The following worksheet will help you obtain the information necessary in making a decision about the consultant's recommendations. The questions are grouped into three separate treatment categories: no treatment, outpatient treatment, and inpatient treatment. Note that several of the questions identified below apply to outpatient and inpatient recommendations.

If No Treatment Alternative Is Recommended

Ask: Do we have a problem then?

Why Ask: If you don't have a problem ... great! But because you have made an investment of time, money, and effort, don't leave the session without a detailed explanation.

Consultant's Answer:

Ask: Even though we don't have a present problem, do you have any suggestions for the future?

Why Ask: Make your investment work for you. Get the professional's recommendations about issues such as prevention and parenting techniques. Use every minute of the session to ask any other questions that relate to your child's needs and your parenting skills.

Consultant's Answer:

If Outpatient Counseling Is Recommended

Ask: Why did you recommend this treatment or program from the continuum of care for my child?

Why Ask: The answer to this question can give you information about your child's present AOD use pattern. You obviously want to do what is necessary to treat the current abuse problem, but you don't want overkill. Make sure that the recommended level of care and resources matches your child's actual needs.

Consultant's Answer:

Ask: Based on your evaluation, does my child have other psychiatric problems in addition to the AOD abuse problem? If so, will these be addressed in the treatment process?

Why Ask: Whether AOD abuse or dependency is a primary disorder or a symptom of other problems is a controversial issue. You want to select a mental health professional or program that bridges the gap between these two opposing viewpoints, one that treats the AOD abuse and behavior as well as the potential emotional problems and issues.

Consultant's Answer:

Ask: What are the credentials and experience of the recommended outpatient therapist?

Why Ask: There are several professional backgrounds to consider: psychiatrists with medical degrees, psychologists with doctorate degrees, social workers, family and marriage counselors with a minimum of a master's degree, and other mental health therapists with a master's degree in an appropriate field. Regardless of the credentials, make sure that each candidate has expertise in child AOD abuse and is a licensed or certified professional in your state. If not, consult another professional.

Consultant's Answer:

Ask: Will our insurance cover this type of treatment? How do we find out?

Why Ask: You need to know the cost of the services recommended for your child. For example, will the costs be covered by a third party? How much will you be required to pay? Will you need to make a cash deposit? Get the answers to these questions to ensure that you select a therapist or treatment program within your budget requirements.

Consultant's Answer:

Ask: How many sessions will this involve?

Why Ask: This can be a tough question to answer on an outpatient basis. Although the number of sessions usually depends on the responses and progress of the client, managed care organizations typically approve only a limited number of outpatient sessions, which is subject to ongoing review.

Consultant's Answer:

Ask: How will our family be involved in our child's treatment?

Why Ask: You should expect an outpatient program to include regularly scheduled family counseling sessions. During this time, you will participate in educational programs, as well as in group and family therapy.

Consultant's Answer:

Ask: What is the success rate for this type of problem?

Why Ask: This is often a great mystery, because most private practitioners and outpatient and inpatient programs do not conduct outcome studies of individual success rates. But ask the question anyway. You or your insurance company may be spending a good deal of money for treatment. For this kind of investment, you deserve a clear and honest response.

Consultant's Answer:

Ask: How will the issue of confidentiality be handled during and after treatment?

Why Ask: The therapist, treatment clinic, or center should agree not to give out any information unless you agree and sign a release. You may also want to consider releasing this information to significant others if it's in your child's best interest.

Consultant's Answer:

If Day, Inpatient, or Residential Treatment Is Recommended

Ask: Why did you recommend this treatment or program for my child?

Why Ask: The answer to this question can give you information about your child's present AOD use pattern. You obviously want to do what is necessary to treat the current abuse problem, but you don't want overkill. Make sure that the recommended level of care and resources matches your child's actual needs.

Consultant's Answer:

Ask: Based on your evaluation, does my child have other psychiatric problems in addition to the AOD abuse problem? If so, will these be addressed in the treatment process?

Why Ask: Whether AOD abuse or dependency is a primary disorder or a symptom of other problems is a controversial issue. You want to select a mental health professional or program that bridges the gap between these two opposing viewpoints, one that treats the AOD abuse and behavior as well as the potential emotional problems and issues.

Consultant's Answer:

Ask: What are the credentials and experience of the members of the recommended treatment team?

Why Ask: A treatment team consists of professionals and staff members with various backgrounds who work with the client and provide their distinct input to the overall treatment effort. The team should be directed by a psychiatrist with a medical degree. Other team members include psychologists with doctorate degrees, registered psychiatric nurses, educators, social workers, and other mental health therapists with a master's degree in an appropriate field. Recovering people are often on the staff under the supervision of a qualified professional. Obtain this information prior to admitting your child to the program.

Consultant's Answer:

Ask: If this treatment is provided in a hospital or residential program, is it approved by the Joint Commission for the Accreditation of Healthcare Organizations (JCAHO)?

Why Ask: This is an absolute necessity. Make sure that the facility and program are accredited by the Joint Commission for the Accreditation of Hospitals (JCAH) or the Commission of Accreditation of Rehabilitation Services or the state. Accept no less under any circumstances.

Consultant's Answer:

Ask: Will our insurance cover this type of treatment? How do we find out?

Why Ask: You need to know the costs of the services recommended for your child. For example, will the costs be covered by a third party? How much will you be required to pay? Will you need to make a cash deposit? Get the answers to these questions to ensure that you select a therapist or treatment program within your budget requirements.

Consultant's Answer:

Ask: How will our family be involved in our child's treatment, including the decision for discharge and the aftercare?

Why Ask: An inpatient program should provide a family component lasting a few days or weekly sessions that continue until the end of treatment. During this time, you will participate in educational programs, as well as in group and family therapy.

Consultant's Answer:

Ask: How will my child continue education while in treatment?

Why Ask: If treatment is expected to last more than a week, you don't want your child to lose school time and risk the consequences. Be sure the inpatient staff includes teachers who will help keep your child current with school work. You will have to sign a release of information form so that teachers in the facility may contact the school to make the arrangements.

Consultant's Answer:

Ask: How will the issue of confidentiality be handled during and after treatment?

Why Ask: The therapist, treatment clinic, or center should agree not to give out any information unless you agree and sign a release. You may also want to consider releasing information to significant others if it's in your child's best interest.

Consultant's Answer:

Ask: How long will the treatment process continue?

Why Ask: This can be a tough question to answer. Often answers depend on the responses and progress of the client. Inpatient programs usually involve a minimum of two weeks, a month, or longer depending on the severity of the problem. But this is rapidly changing. Managed care companies no longer accept this. Instead, they approve limited number of sessions, which is subject to ongoing review. Also, the admission standards for treatment are more rigorous. Find out about this and weigh the information, taking into account your insurance and overall budget considerations.

Consultant's Answer:

Ask: When my child is discharged from this phase of treatment, how will it be decided what types of ongoing treatment will be necessary?

Why Ask: An effective treatment program should have continuing care consisting of weekly peer group support sessions that last one to two years after inpatient treatment. The program should also include group therapy, ongoing referral to other self-help groups, and follow-up contact with clients on a regular basis, tracking their progress to ensure a successful re-entry into the community.

Consultant's Answer:

Ask: What is the program's success rate? Are statistics available that define the social, emotional, and physical growth or improvement of clients?

Why Ask: This can be a great mystery because most private practitioners and outpatient and inpatient programs do not conduct outcome studies of individual success rates. But ask the question anyway. You or your insurance company may be spending a good deal of money for treatment. For this kind of investment, you deserve a clear and honest response.

Consultant's Answer:

Following the Recommendations

If you accept the professional's recommendations, use the guidelines below to select the most appropriate strategy.

- If no AOD or other serious problems exist and your child is between the ages of 5 and 10, use Strategy 1 on page 19. Although you have no current problem, this strategy will provide information and the structure to help prevent future AOD abuse by your child.
- If no AOD or other serious problems exist and your child is between the ages of 9 and 13, use Strategy 2 on page 41. Although you have no current problem, this strategy will provide information and the structure to help prevent future AOD abuse by your child.
- If outpatient counseling is recommended, use Strategy 4 on page 75.
- If a change in the home environment is recommended, use Strategy 5 on page 77.
- If an intervention is recommended, use Strategy 6 on page 97.
- If inpatient or residential treatment is recommended, use Strategy 7 on page 101.

Strategy 4

Knowing What to Expect from Outpatient Counseling

Usually, the consulting professional will be the outpatient counselor. But if this is not the case, select a counselor using the criteria established in Strategy 3. When working with the counselor, expect that your rights, responsibilities, and integrity will be affirmed. You will be respected as caregivers concerned about the overall well-being of your child. If you are a loving, caring, and responsible parent and/or caregiver seeking professional guidance, do not believe that poor skills on your part caused the present circumstance. At no time should you feel like you are being judged.

Too often caregivers fall into a guilt trip that makes it difficult to address the real issue behind their child's choice to use alcohol or other drugs (AOD). At the first session, use the same worksheets you did with the consultation professional. If the consultant is now your therapist, this point is moot. If you are working with another counseling professional, however, the questions will help you determine your satisfaction with the counselor and the course of treatment.

If you have not done so, review your responses to the Evaluation Inventory (page 3) and "High-Risk Factors for AOD Abuse Questionnaire" (page 16) with the counselor prior to the first counseling session with your child. Your input may be of assistance to the counselor. After all, depending solely on input from the child is unwise because children and teenagers underestimate, deny, or distort the reality of their AOD abuse. Although skilled counselors are prepared for excuses, manipulation, scapegoating, or exaggeration by their clients, your perspective as the child's guardian will give the professional a head start in the evaluation of your child. The results of your evaluation will also provide the counselor valuable information on how your child feels about his AOD use, who your child describes as her peers and what activities they prefer, why your child drinks or uses drugs, how your child uses AOD, and what the consequences of your child's AOD abuse may be.

If this strategy is successful, use Strategy 1 or 2 to obtain information and develop the structure to help prevent future AOD abuse by your child. You may have tried one of these strategies earlier. But because outpatient counseling has been effective, you are now in a position to use a prevention plan.

There is a possibility the therapist will recommend a more structured family approach, such as the one described in Strategy 5. If not, ask the counselor if Strategy 5 should be used in conjunction with counseling. But don't use this strategy on your own without professional input. It is designed to be used in the context of the other strategies and counseling to be effective. If you've used a structured home environment in conjunction with outpatient counseling and your child chooses to continue his AOD abuse, intervention or inpatient/residential treatment may be necessary. Do not expect overnight success or an instant miracle. Your child's AOD abuse pattern and problems did not develop overnight. Consequently, counseling will take time and patience to resolve and eliminate your child's AOD abuse.

Strategy 5

Designing the Structured Home Environment: Expectations, Choices, and Consequences

Preaching and teaching about the horrors of addiction or the evils of alcohol are generally ineffective as prevention measures. In addition, coercing children to avoid using AOD has shown little success. Children will listen to a theory but usually will not heed the messages about AOD abuse, regardless of the logic, reason, or truth. To effectively confront and stop your child's AOD abuse, the structured home environment strategy provides you with a practical, step-by-step process. It should only be used in conjunction with consultation or outpatient counseling recommendations.

The strategy uses a trial-and-error process and common-sense approach, based on the idea that experience is the best teacher. Its purpose is two-fold. First, it will show your child that AOD abuse has a logical and predictable pattern leading to pain and unpleasantness. Second, it will motivate your child to consider a different, more constructive lifestyle without abusing AOD. You'll learn how to implement a ten-step process to make your child more accountable and responsible for her behavior. You will discover what to expect from your child when using this strategy and how to respond. In addition, you will learn what to do if your child continues abusing AOD.

How the Ten-Step Process Works

1. **You should determine expectations for your child.** Examples to consider include the following:
   - When should curfew be set?
   - What household chores should we assign?
   - What should we expect about homework?
   - School grades?
   - What is reasonable behavior?
   - How much do we give for an allowance?
   - What is our policy about friends in the house?
   - Phone calls?

- Are AOD off limits?

Why? You should take the time to determine reasonable expectations for your child. Although your primary concern is AOD abuse, the learning by mistakes and trial-and-error process should include as many expectations as you can generate. The no AOD use rule should be just one of the general expectations.

2. **You and your significant other should both agree with the expectations.**

   Why? If you as the parents and caregivers of the child are not unified, then your child may exploit the situation and pursue the easier adult or most convenient rule. As a result, your child will be able to manipulate you, evade the primary issue of personal responsibility, and not learn by mistakes. Before talking to your child, make sure you and your significant other resolve your differences concerning reasonable expectations.

3. **If you are a single parent, be firm and confident with the reasons and fairness of the expectations.**

   Why? Your child will perceive your hesitation about expectations and may be less inclined to follow the rules.

4. **Present and explain the expectations to your child.**

   Why? A fundamental part of structuring the family, this will be important when you discuss choices and consequences later in the process. Take time to sit down with your child and carefully, confidently, and clearly present the expectations. Do it even if you believe your child knows the rules and will break them anyway.

5. **Make sure that the child understands the expectations.**

   Why? This will prevent any excuses or claims by your child that he was not aware of a particular rule. Do not give your child this opportunity to manipulate you or use ignorance as an alibi for his conduct.

6. **Do not compromise any expectations where the use of AOD is involved.**

   Why? A child should not use AOD other than for legitimate medical or religious reasons. At all times, be reasonable, firm, and consistent about this. Do not compromise or negotiate any issues regarding the use of AOD and certainly do not teach your child how to use illegal AOD in moderation. A judge would never understand this rationale.

7. **Reach an agreement with your child about the expectations.**

   Why? If your child does not agree with a particular expectation, discuss the disagreement. You might even consider a reasonable alternative except where

AOD are involved. If your child refuses to agree by word and deed, you should consider a serious consequence. A child who will not obey your rules is out of control and requires immediate corrective action. Your child should understand this point of view.

8. **Explain to your child that if she doesn't follow expectations, it will be her choice.**

   Why? You want to give her the opportunity to make her own decisions and choices. If she chooses to follow the expectations, she will earn praise, encouragement, trust, and responsibility. Ideally, if she practices this pattern long enough, following the expectations may become second nature. This may increase the likelihood she will stop using AOD. Impress upon your child, without begging or pleading, that she has the freedom and opportunity to make choices.

9. **Make sure that your child understands that if she chooses not to follow an expectation, consequences will follow.**

   Why? Allow your child to decide upon her own consequences. Put the emphasis on the choices, not the consequences. After all, this is a reality of life. It applies to everyone. If your child makes enough bad decisions with unpleasant consequences, perhaps she will become motivated to consider a more constructive alternative.

10. **If your child chooses not to follow expectations, use progressively enforceable consequences with restrictions on things your child values.**

    Example 1: If your child chooses not to follow expectations or uses AOD, he volunteers to

    - forfeit the use of the car if old enough,
    - be confined to his room without television or the stereo,
    - not attend a rock concert for two months, or
    - be "grounded" or restricted from social activities with his friends for two weeks.

    Example 2: If your child chooses not to come home at a specific time, restrict his outside social activities for a week. If he chooses again not to come home at the predesignated time, restrict his outside social activities for two or three weeks.

    Why? If your child experiences the progressive degrees of unpleasantness resulting from his choice not to follow expectations, he may be motivated to consider a different, more constructive lifestyle. If your child continues to ignore expectations, he is volunteering to give up the stereo, telephone, television, or time spent with friends—all things children don't want to live without. Ask your child why he chooses to deprive himself of things he likes. Remember that you are giving your child an opportunity to learn by his mistakes. His mistakes will only result in undesirable consequences. Unfortunately, your child's behavior may result in an arrest for a juvenile offense such as incorrigibility, possession of an illegal substance, runaway, curfew violation, or truancy.

As hard as it may seem, try to make the best of a bad situation. You need not fear court intervention, which can serve as an ultimate consequence of your child's continued, repeated choice to abuse AOD and laws. Actually, some parents and caregivers become so frustrated with the child's continued negative behaviors that they seek court intervention. Because children can place blame on their caregivers rather than accept blame for their own actions, however, this can be a premature overreaction that lessens the impact of the court intervention. Your child should ultimately volunteer for court intervention as a result of his repeated negative behaviors. Unless your child commits a crime or poses a danger to himself or others that would require immediate court intervention, prevention, detection, and counseling efforts should be initiated prior to court intervention.

Knowing What to Expect from Your Child and How to Respond

Children who consistently abuse AOD will often develop an incorrigible thought and behavior pattern in a short period of time. For this reason, you can expect that your child will resist a structured home environment, especially because it now has expectations, choices, and consequences. Trying to discuss issues in a direct, yet respectful, calm demeanor when your child reacts angrily will be a challenge. As difficult as it may be, though, you should use the opportunity to teach him to clarify his remarks, improve his logic, and change his behavior. This is, no doubt, an awesome task, but the following pages can help ease the burden.

Identified below are a number of typical reactions you may expect from your child about the expectations, choices, and consequences as well as other issues with this structure. Included are the most practical, effective ways for you to respond. Review the following examples to understand the statement-response pattern and use them on a consistent basis. Note that several of your responses may be used repeatedly with different reactions.

When your child: Tells you why she should not be held accountable for her choices that led to the particular mess she is in.

You: Listen to reasonable explanations, but accept no excuses. Do not discuss why's of the issue. Tell her that rationalizations are irrelevant and another way for her to avoid the problem. Give her examples of her faulty logic on this matter and show her how to change her behavior. Keep the focus and discussion on the real issue: her irresponsible choices.

When your child: Insists that he has rights, not responsibilities, and his rights are always being violated.

You: Listen to reasonable explanations, but accept no excuses. Do not discuss why's of the issue. Tell him that rationalizations are irrelevant and another way for him to avoid the problem. Give him examples of his faulty logic on this matter and show him how to change his behavior. Keep the focus and discussion on the real issue: his irresponsible choices.

When your child: Thinks she is different and better than others.

You: Discuss why her logic doesn't make sense. Give her examples of her faulty logic on this matter and show her how to change her behavior. Help her examine her assumptions and how they defy the facts. Keep the focus and discussion on the real issue: her irresponsible choices.

When your child: Bases his decisions on assumptions, not facts.

You: Discuss why his logic doesn't make sense. Help him examine his assumptions and understand how they defy the facts. Help him understand the facts.

When your child: Uses and possesses people and objects.

You: Call attention to her attempts to use you and others by saying, "I don't like it when you try to manipulate me." Then explain that you know when you're being used. Tell her when she is using control and manipulation over others. Point out the differences between legitimate control and persuasion as opposed to manipulation and exploitation. Reverse the circumstances and ask her how she would feel if treated this way.

When your child: Fakes dependence to take advantage of a person or situation.

You: Listen to reasonable explanations, but accept no excuses. Tell him when he is using control and manipulation over others. Call attention to his attempts to use you and others by saying, "I don't like it when you try to manipulate me." Then explain that you know when you're being used. Keep the focus and discussion on the real issue: his irresponsible choices.

When your child: Practices denial and uses a myriad of defense mechanisms such as projection, rationalization, minimization, and blame to explain and excuse her behavior.

You: Listen to reasonable explanations, but accept no excuses. Discuss why her logic doesn't make sense. Do not discuss why's of the issue. Tell her that rationalizations are irrelevant and another way for her to avoid the problem. Keep the focus and discussion on the real issue: her irresponsible choices.

When your child: Is vague, silent, and secretive, believing power exists in secrecy.

You: Give him examples of his faulty logic on this matter and show him how to change his behavior. Describe how he uses his selective memory and is able to remember only what he wants. Tell him when he is using control and manipulation over others. Call attention to his attempts to use you and others by saying, "I don't like it when you try to manipulate me." Then explain that you know when you're being used.

When your child: Blames others and society for her predicament and claims she's a helpless, innocent victim.

You: Listen to reasonable explanations, but accept no excuses. Do not discuss why's of the issue. Tell her that rationalizations are irrelevant and another way for her to avoid the problem. Give her examples of her faulty logic on this matter and show her how to change her behavior. Keep the focus and discussion on the real issue: her irresponsible choices.

When your child: Resists recommendations for work, school, or any other normal tasks and functions because they bore him.

You: Listen to reasonable explanations, but accept no excuses. Do not accept unreasonable "I can't" statements. Often "I can't" means "I won't" or "I don't want to." Explain that making an effort sometimes means doing what you don't want to do. Point out that he usually has more than enough energy to do what he wants to do. In a nonthreatening manner, explain that negative consequences may result from lack of effort.

When your child: Says "I can't," which otherwise means that she won't.

You: Listen to reasonable explanations, but accept no excuses. Do not accept "I can't" statements. Understand that "I can't" means "I won't" and usually involves doing what she does not feel like doing. Explain that making an effort sometimes means doing what you don't want to do. Point out that she usually has more than enough energy to do what she wants to do.

When your child: Expects immediate success.

You: Try to get him to identify his expectations. Discuss why his logic doesn't make sense. Help him examine his assumptions and understand how they defy the facts. Teach him that success usually doesn't happen overnight. Point out that immediate decisions may not work as planned. Use examples to show that we all make mistakes, but we can learn from them. Describe it as trial by error. Help him accept the disappointment of failure in a constructive way.

When your child: Quits at the first sign of failure.

You: Listen to reasonable explanations, but accept no excuses. Point out that effort sometimes means doing what you don't want to do. Point out that she has plenty of energy for things that she wants to do. In a nonthreatening manner, explain that negative consequences may result from lack of effort. Use examples to show that we all make mistakes, but we can learn from them. Describe it as trial by error.

When your child: Expects others to immediately respond to his demands.

You: Give him examples of his faulty logic on this matter and show him how to change his behavior. Tell him when he is using control and manipulation over others. Call attention to his attempts to use you and others by saying, "I don't like it when you try to manipulate me." Then explain that you know when you're being used.

When your child: Has a compelling need to be in control of every situation.

You: Give her examples of her faulty logic on this matter and show her how to change her behavior. Tell her when she is using control and manipulation over others. Call attention to her attempts to use you and others by saying, "I don't like it when you try to manipulate me." Then explain that you know when you're being used. Point out the differences between legitimate control and persuasion as opposed to manipulation and exploitation.

When your child: Uses manipulation and deceit.

You: Give him examples of his faulty logic on this matter and show him how to change his behavior. Tell him when he is using control and manipulation over others. Call attention to his attempts to use you and others by saying, "I don't like it when you try to manipulate me." Then explain that you know when you're being used.

When your child: Appears not to listen or believes you're wasting her time.

You: Tell her when she is using control and manipulation over others. Call attention to her attempts to use you and others by saying, "I don't like it when you try to manipulate me." Then explain that you know when you're being used. Point out the differences between legitimate control and persuasion as opposed to manipulation and exploitation. Keep the focus and discussion on the real issue: her irresponsible choices.

When your child: Will not consider doing what you ask others to do.

You: Listen to reasonable explanations, but accept no excuses. Point that out he has plenty of energy for things that he wants to do. In a nonthreatening manner, explain that negative consequences may result from no effort. Do not accept "I can't" statements. Understand that "I can't" means "I won't" and usually involves doing what he does not feel like doing.

Contracting with Your Child

Make contracts with your child to implement and use expectations, choices, and consequences. The two sample contract formats on the following pages illustrate how this may be accomplished. Use either format or make changes appropriate for your situation. Keep in mind the following ten-step process while reviewing each of the formats.

1. You should determine expectations for your child.
2. You and your significant other should both agree with the expectations.
3. If you are a single parent, be firm and confident with the reasons and fairness of the expectations.
4. Present and explain the expectations to your child.
5. Make sure that the child understands the expectations.
6. Do not compromise any expectations where the use of AOD is involved.
7. Reach an agreement with your child about the expectations.
8. Explain to your child that if she doesn't follow expectations, it will be her choice.
9. Make sure that your child understands that if she chooses not to follow an expectation, consequences will follow.
10. If your child chooses not to follow expectations, use progressively enforceable consequences with restrictions on things your child values.

Sample Contract #1

Name of Child: ______________________________

I am changing my lifestyle. I will not go to the following places:

1. ______________________________

2. ______________________________

I am changing my friends. These are the people I will not call or see:

1. ______________________________

2. ______________________________

If I call or see any of the above people, I will accept the following consequences:

1. ______________________________

2. ______________________________

These are the friends and acquaintances I will spend time with:

1. ______________________________

2. ______________________________

These are the times I am setting for myself:

1. I will be in the house at ____________________ Sundays through Thursdays.
2. I will be in the house at ____________________ Fridays and Saturdays.
3. I will be awake and out of bed at ____________________ on weekdays.
4. I will be awake and out of bed at ____________________ on weekends.

If I am irresponsible and don't follow these guidelines, these will be my consequences:

1. ______________________________

2. ______________________________

When I go out, I will inform my parents/caregivers:

1. Where I am going or getting permission to go
2. What I intend to do
3. Who is providing transportation

4. What people I will be with

5. When I plan to return

I will call if I change locations.

If I have to go out before my parent(s)/caregiver(s) return home, I will leave a note as to my whereabouts and approximate time of return.

I will place a calendar of all upcoming events in a prominent place. If I do not follow the above requirements, these are my consequences:

1. ______________________________

2. ______________________________

The following jobs at home must be completed before I am entitled to any privileges:

1. Daily __________ Weekly __________ As Needed __________

2. Daily __________ Weekly __________ As Needed __________

I will not need to be reminded and will do my work thoroughly. If I do not follow through with the above agreement, these are my consequences:

1. ______________________________

2. ______________________________

SIGNED:

Child ______________________________

Date ______________________________

Parent(s)/Caregiver(s) ______________________________

Parent(s)/Caregiver(s) ______________________________

Sample Contract #2

This contract is between ____________________ and Child Parent(s)/Caregiver(s)

General Expectations

The Use of Alcohol and Other Illegal Drugs

Expectations

1. ____________________ By When: ____________
2. ____________________ By When: ____________
3. ____________________ By When: ____________

Consequences

1. ____________________
2. ____________________
3. ____________________

Rewards

1. ____________________
2. ____________________
3. ____________________

Bedroom

Expectations

1. ____________________ By When: ____________
2. ____________________ By When: ____________
3. ____________________ By When: ____________

Consequences

1. ____________________
2. ____________________
3. ____________________

Rewards

1. ______________________________
2. ______________________________
3. ______________________________

Kitchen

Expectations

1. ____________________ By When: ____________
2. ____________________ By When: ____________
3. ____________________ By When: ____________

Consequences

1. ______________________________
2. ______________________________
3. ______________________________

Rewards

1. ______________________________
2. ______________________________
3. ______________________________

Bathroom

Expectations

1. ____________________ By When: ____________
2. ____________________ By When: ____________
3. ____________________ By When: ____________

Consequences

1. ______________________________
2. ______________________________
3. ______________________________

Rewards

1. ______________________________

2. ______________________________

3. ______________________________

Yard and Garage

Expectations

1. ____________________ By When: ____________

2. ____________________ By When: ____________

3. ____________________ By When: ____________

Consequences

1. ______________________________

2. ______________________________

3. ______________________________

Rewards

1. ______________________________

2. ______________________________

3. ______________________________

Phone Privileges

Expectations

1. Daily phone calls are limited to the hours of ____________ P.M.

2. No calls will be received after ____________ P.M.

3. Parents/caregivers will answer the phone after ____________ P.M.

4. ______________________________

Consequences

1. ______________________________

2. ______________________________

3. ______________________________

Rewards

1. ______________________________

2. ______________________________

3. ______________________________

School Requirements

Expectations

1. I will attend all classes and complete all assignments.

2. If I have no homework, I will read for ______________________________.

3. ______________________________

Consequences

1. ______________________________

2. ______________________________

3. ______________________________

Rewards

1. ______________________________

2. ______________________________

3. ______________________________

Use of Car

Expectations

1. ______________________________

2. ______________________________

3. ______________________________

Consequences

1. ______________________________

2. ______________________________

3. ______________________________

Rewards

1. ______________________________

2. ______________________________

3. ______________________________

Curfew

Expectations

1. Weeknights (Sunday through Thursday) I am to be home by ____________ P.M.

2. Weekends (Friday and Saturday) I am to be home by ____________ P.M.

3. Curfew will only be extended by special request in advance at the discretion of the parents or caregivers.

4. Privilege nights are ______________________________

5. ______________________________

Consequences

1. ______________________________

2. ______________________________

3. ______________________________

Rewards

1. ______________________________

2. ______________________________

3. ______________________________

Attitude and Language

Expectations

1. I will treat my parents/caregivers with respect. I will treat family members, guests, and parents/caregivers as they wish to be treated.

2. I will not use foul language around the house.

3. I will not slam doors, hit walls, or throw temper tantrums.

4. I will not shout at people who get in my way.

Consequences

1. ______________________________

2. ______________________________

3. ______________________________

Rewards

1. ______________________________

2. ______________________________

3. ______________________________

Failure to meet the requirements of this contract including any use of AOD will result in:

1. Counseling

2. Treatment

3. Legal intervention

4. Other ______________________________

This contract will be reviewed and if necessary, renegotiated by both parties on or before ____________. We, the undersigned, understand and agree to abide by the conditions of this contract.

Dated ______________________________

Parent(s)/Caregiver(s) ______________________________

Parent(s)/Caregiver(s) ______________________________

Child ______________________________

Counselor/Therapist ______________________________

Understanding What Not to Do with Your Child

- Do not make "empty" threats that you cannot enforce.

  Why? Expectations and consequences are only effective if you are prepared to back them up.

  If your child says: I'm going to do it and you can't stop me," or "I'm not going to do it. Just try and make me."

  Don't say: "You do and you'll be sorry," or "If you don't, you're going to get it."

  Instead say: "That will be your choice and you know the consequences." Then be prepared to give the consequences based on his choice.

- Do not give your child money for any reason other than legitimate expenses.

  Why? The money might otherwise be used to buy AOD.

  If your child says: "I lost my lunch money again," or "I need $5 for a school project."

  Don't say: "Okay. Here it is," or "No way." Rather, determine if the request is justifiable.

  Instead say: "You need to be more careful with your money," or "In the future, let me know sooner."

- Do not nag your child about her AOD abuse.

  Why? Actions speak louder than words. If your child chooses to abuse AOD, let her worry about the consequences.

  If your child says: "You can count on it. I'm not going to drink."

  Don't say: "You'd better not drink or if you get caught by the cops, you'll spend the night in jail. Don't count on me to bail you out." Those words will have little effect on her choice.

  Instead say: "If you drink, that will be your choice and you know the consequences." Then be prepared to give the consequences based on her choice.

- Do not accept obnoxious, offensive, or destructive behavior by your child as normal.

  Why? You will lose your perspective and sense of objectivity. Ultimately, you may rely too much on emotions and overreact to the situation.

  If your child says: "You can't stop me," "Try and make me," or "Drop dead," or if he threatens you.

Don't say: "Watch your step, young man," or "Keep it up and you're going to get it."

Instead say: "That will be your choice and you know the consequences." Then be prepared to give the consequences based on his choice. This may include contacting the police if you are threatened physically.

- Do not confront your child with questions or consequences if he is under the influence of AOD.

  Why? It will be like talking to a statue or even worse, he may become unnecessarily angry or violent. Wait to talk with him until the effects have worn off.

  If your child says: "Leave me alone," "Get out of my life," or "I just want to go to bed."

  Don't say: "You've had it," "This is your last warning," or "Look at me when I'm talking to you."

  Instead say: "We'll discuss this when you're sober." Then be prepared to give the consequences based on his choice.

- Do not make excuses to anyone about your child's AOD abuse.

  Why? Your child is responsible for her AOD abuse. She must face the reality of her abuse and by excusing the behavior, you prolong reality.

  If your child says: "You've got to help me or I'll get kicked out of school for drinking."

  Don't say: "I'll help you this time, but you have to promise never to do anything like this again."

  Instead say: "I can't lie for you. You made the choice, so be prepared to accept the consequence. Perhaps you will learn from your mistake."

- Do not take responsibility for your child's AOD-related problems.

  Why? If your child knows that you will bail him out or assume the responsibility, he will be denied the experience of solving his own problems. Obviously, the AOD abuse will continue if there is no consequence.

  If your child says: "You've got to help me or I'll get busted for possession of pot."

  Don't say: "I'll help you this time, but you have to promise never to do anything like this again."

  Instead say: "I can't lie for you. You made the choice, be prepared to accept the consequence. Perhaps you will be able to learn from your mistake."

- Do not solve your child's problems that result from her choice to abuse AOD.

  Why? Your child needs to experience the results to truly understand what happens when she chooses to abuse AOD. The more unpleasant or painful the results, the more desirable it becomes to stop the AOD abuse and seek positive alternatives or help for the abuse problem.

  If your child says: "I need money to pay my court fees for the possession conviction."

  Don't say: "I'll pay the money this time, but you have to promise never to do anything like this again."

  Instead say: "I will loan you the money, but you will need to pay it back. You made the choice, so be prepared to accept the consequence. Perhaps you will be able to learn from your mistake."

- Do not wish away the problem or patronize your child in the hope that he will suddenly see the light and stop abusing AOD.

  Why? Wishing or hoping will NOT make the problem disappear. Instead, be prepared for excuses, promises of change, arguments that it's no big deal, or efforts to change the subject.

  If your child says: "I don't want to talk about it," "I don't have a problem," or "I promise I'll never drink again."

  Don't say: "You do and you'll be sorry," or "If you don't, you're going to get it."

  Instead say: "That will be your choice and you know the consequences." Then be prepared to give the consequences based on his choice.

- Do not let your child's behavior adversely affect your attitude and behavior.

  Why? Your child will find it more difficult to resist firmness, objectivity, and your perspective.

  If your child says: "You can't stop me," or "Try and make me."

  Don't say: "You do and you'll be sorry," or "If you don't, you're going to get it."

  Instead say: "That will be your choice and you know the consequences." Then be prepared to give the consequences based on his choice.

- Do not assume that your child does not love you.

  Why? The natural, predictable effects of AOD abuse are delusion, confusion, and self-guilt. The AOD abuser simply cannot love or care about anyone.

If your child says: "I hate you and everything you stand for," "I can't wait to get away from you," or "You're going to wake up one day and I'll be gone."

Don't say: "You'll be sorry for saying that," or "One day, you'll thank me for this."

Instead say: "That will be your choice and you know the consequences." Then be prepared to continue to give consequences based on his choice.

- Do not conclude that your child lacks willpower or that expectations, choices, and consequences are not working.

  Why? Your child's energy and willpower are directed toward a destructive goal. Although each individual is unique and can endure more or less unpleasantness than the next person, most of us have a threshold that triggers surrender. In this case, surrender does not mean giving up, but rather, giving in to avoid giving up on life.

Remember, if the child has the opportunity to experience the unpleasant results of his substance abuse, it is logical to assume that the teen will be motivated to consider a different, more constructive lifestyle or alternatives to AOD abuse. Instead, be prepared to help your child get help.

Just in Case

By now, your knowledge about child or teen AOD abuse is more advanced than most parents and other caregivers. Knowledge is only one part of the puzzle in stopping your child's AOD abuse, however. Your child may still resist change, which may mean that she's extensively involved in AOD abuse. If the use of a structured home environment in conjunction with outpatient counseling is unsuccessful, intervention will be necessary. In fact, your outpatient counselor may recommend it anyway.

Strategy 6

Understanding How and When to Use the Intervention Process

Intervention may be necessary to put your child in touch with the reality of his condition and the need for help. With this strategy, you will learn how the intervention process works and how to do it step by step. Intervention is a process used by parents and other caregivers to confront the AOD-abusing child with the reality of her condition. In this situation, the objective is to make her aware of the need for help and provide her with treatment options. How a person gets to this point is due to what people in Alcoholics Anonymous refer to as the "cunning, powerful, and baffling" addiction process.

During the addiction process, a person builds a remarkable alibi or denial system. To defend and protect her AOD abuse, she shuns the real world by using such defense mechanisms as rationalization, projection, manipulation, and avoidance. Other defense mechanisms include minimizing ("It's no big deal." "It's not that bad."); avoiding the subject (ignoring or refusing to talk about the problem or distracting others from the subject); absolute denying ("I can stop anytime." "No, I don't have a problem." "How can a behavior be addicting?"); and blaming others ("My parents, friends, and teachers are driving me nuts." "I do it, but so would anybody else in my situation.").

Her denial system may be additionally reinforced by the following:

- **Chemically induced blackouts.** In this case, the child suffers from memory lapses, or blackouts, while under the influence of AOD. Because of this, she can't recall her specific feelings at the time or her resulting bizarre, destructive, and antisocial behavior.
- **Psychologically induced blackouts.** The child represses remorseful feelings like guilt and shame. She literally shuts out these feelings and thereby rationalizes her bizarre behavior caused by the AOD abuse.
- **Euphoric recall.** The child remembers the good times and feelings when using AOD but conveniently fails to recollect how she behaved under the influence. This process also helps her forget her present physical, social, and emotional pain and unpleasantness.

Given the natural evolution of the addiction process and the denial system, you should know and accept the painful truth that your child does not have the willpower or fortitude to stop her use of AOD and/or has developed a denial system to defend her use of AOD because she is either unwilling or unable to objectively perceive or understand the reality of her condition

When to Use the Intervention Process

The intervention process should be used when the combination of prevention measures, professional counseling efforts, and a structured home environment has been unsuccessful in stopping your child's AOD abuse, or when a professional counselor has evaluated your child's AOD abuse pattern and made a determination of AOD dependency.

If your outpatient counselor is not able to help you with the intervention, then select a professional who has expertise and experience in using the intervention process for child or teen AOD abuse and dependency. Ask for referrals from a trusted friends who has experienced a similar situation, your family physician, your community's mental health association, or your community's mental health center. Once you have a list of qualified professionals, call each one and ask questions about how to handle your specific situation. Then select a professional who seems most able to help.

Who Is Involved in the Intervention Process

The intervention process is a team effort consisting of two or more participants who play an important role in the child's life: the parent(s) or caregiver(s); family members and significant others close to the child who have witnessed his strange, antisocial, AOD-related behavior; and the professional counselor with expertise and experience in the intervention of child or teen AOD abuse and dependency

How Your Step-by-Step Intervention Plan of Action Works

1. **Arrange a consultation with a professional counselor with expertise in childhood and adolescent AOD abuse, dependency, and the intervention process.** The professional will be present at the intervention with your child to coordinate the proceedings. At the consultation, review the efforts you have made to stop your child's AOD abuse, cite the documented AOD-related behaviors of your child, identify other meaningful people close to your child who have witnessed her AOD-related behaviors and are willing to be participants in the intervention, determine a date to review the information and logistics with all participants except your child, and identify a recent crisis, or

several crises, involving your child's AOD-related behavior. Usually, the most suitable time for the intervention is as soon as possible after the crisis. Examples of such a crisis are

- being suspended or expelled from school for AOD-related behaviors,
- making verbal threats or engaging in actual physical altercations while under the influence of AOD,
- being in an AOD-related accident, or
- being arrested for drunken driving or public intoxication.

2. **After your consultation, contact the members you have selected for the intervention team.** Request their help for the intervention effort. If they accept, set a meeting time to have the professional discuss the logistics of the intervention with them. All participants should understand the nature of AOD abuse and dependency, the denial system, and the purpose of the intervention.
3. **Each team member should prepare a written list of the AOD-related behaviors of your child.** The list must be detailed and accurate regarding dates, places, and behaviors.
4. **Set the intervention date.** It is essential for your child to be sober and unaware of the intervention date.
5. The professional will coordinate the intervention and direct each team member to objectively point out that:
    - A crisis or several crises have occurred due to your child's AOD abuse.
    - The AOD abuse has caused her extreme emotional, social, and or physical harm.
    - Other people are aware of her problem and want her to seek treatment.
    - If she does not seek treatment, there will be further consequences. Although this is not the time or place to mention this, one other consequence may have to be involuntary commitment to a treatment facility.
    - Her present pain and feelings of anger, remorse, and shame are caused by AOD abuse.
6. Be prepared for an angry, defensive reaction from your child. She will probably use accusations, manipulation, deceit, and resentment to break down the objective, united front of the participants. If the team members are informed, confident, and composed to weather the stormy reaction of your child, however, the chance for a successful intervention is excellent.

7. **Your child's acceptance of an AOD problem and her motivation to seek assistance are crucial to the prospect for recovery.** Even if your child's apparent motivation may be exaggerated and you think she's faking it, discuss what specific types of changes she will need to make to stop her AOD abuse.
8. Let your child choose the type of treatment she would like to pursue including one or more of the following:
   - individual counseling;
   - family and group counseling;
   - support group involvement, such as Alcoholics Anonymous; or
   - inpatient/residential treatment.
9. Although your child may select options A, B, or C, you and your child must agree on one point. If treatment with those options is unsuccessful and she begins to use AOD again, she will risk the possibility of a legal intervention—or you may have no choice but to commit her to an inpatient or residential treatment facility. This is the time to make sure that your child understands the legal and social ramifications if she discontinues or refuses treatment.
10. Be prepared to arrange immediate treatment dates for your child. Individual, family and group sessions and support group meetings should be scheduled. Also, be ready, if necessary, to take steps toward your child's admission to an inpatient or residential treatment program. If intervention is successful, one of 3 strategies will be recommended: 4, 5, or 7. Which strategy you select will be determined at the conclusion of the intervention based on the responses of your child and the recommendation of the attending professional. If this intervention is unsuccessful or if your child is out of control, almost dysfunctional and risking his life and the lives of others by abusing AOD, the last alternative is Strategy 7, involuntary commitment to an inpatient or residential treatment program.

Strategy 7

Selecting an Effective Inpatient/ Residential Treatment Program

If your child is out of control, dysfunctional, and risky with his life and the lives of others by abusing AOD, commitment to an inpatient or residential treat ment program may be necessary. Using this strategy, you will learn how to select the best and most appropriate type of treatment facility to meet your needs and what to expect before, during and after treatment. Your options include the following:

1. **Inpatient hospitalization.** The patients receive comprehensive psychiatric treatment in a hospital. The length of treatment ranges from a few days for acute care and up to 30 days for intermediate care.
2. **A crisis residence.** This setting provides short-term crisis intervention, acute stabilization, detoxification services, and treatment usually for fewer than 15 days. Patients receive 24-hour-per-day supervision.
3. **A residential treatment facility.** Seriously disturbed patients receive intensive and comprehensive psychiatric treatment in a campuslike setting on a long-term basis. If you have to use this strategy, your child most likely has a dependency on AOD. He is both psychologically and physically hooked. Even so, this strategy should be used only in specific circumstances:
   - The combination of prevention measures, professional counseling efforts, and a structured home environment has been unsuccessful in stopping your child's AOD abuse.
   - Your intervention has been successful and your child has accepted the need for help. If your child has not accepted the need for treatment, the alternative may be an involuntary commitment, particularly if he is a danger to himself or others.

   If your child is out of control and poses a danger to herself and others, she may be qualified to receive third party reimbursement. If this is not the case, you will probably have to pay for this expense. Use the questions on the following worksheet to obtain information so that you can make the best decision for your child.

Selection Worksheet

Ask: Does the program have a well-defined treatment philosophy that has been implemented on a practical and logical basis?

Why Ask: One of your first concerns is to find out if the staff involved with the program is qualified. If so, they should be able to give you a comprehensive, understandable mission statement that defines what they do and how they do it. Make sure you see and hear about it.

Consultant's Answer:

Ask: Does the program provide consideration for the special needs of AOD abusing young people? For example, such factors as a child's use of multiple drugs, youth values, and other topics relevant to the child's world should be addressed through counseling, education and group discussions.

Why Ask: You don't want to put your child in a treatment program with adult patients who have nothing in common with the values and needs of young people. Working with adult patients in individual and group therapy sessions and discussions will most likely turn off your child. Only consider a program that addresses and meets the needs of children with AOD-related problems.

Consultant's Answer:

Ask: Based on your evaluation, does my child have other psychiatric problems in addition to the AOD abuse problem? If so, will these be addressed in the treatment process?

Why Ask: Whether AOD abuse or dependency is a primary disorder or a symptom of other problems is a controversial issue. You want to select a program that bridges the gap between these two opposing viewpoints, one that treats the AOD abuse and behavior and the potential emotional problems and issues.

Consultant's Answer:

Ask: What are the credentials and experience of the members of the recommended treatment team?

Why Ask: A treatment team consists of professionals and staff members with various backgrounds who work with the client and provide their input to the treatment effort. The team should be directed by a psychiatrist with a medical degree. Other team members include psychologists with doctorate degrees, registered psychiatric nurses, educators, social workers, family and marriage counselors with a minimum of a master's degree, and other mental health therapists with a master's degree in an appropriate field. Sometimes people on the staff are recovering alcoholics or addicts under the supervision of a qualified professional. Obtain this information before admitting your child to the program.

Consultant's Answer:

Ask: If this treatment is provided in a hospital or residential program, is it approved by the Joint Commission for the Accreditation of Healthcare Organizations (JCAHO)?

Why Ask: This is an absolute necessity. Make sure that the facility and program are accredited by the Joint Commission for the Accreditation of Hospitals (JCAH) or the Commission of Accreditation of Rehabilitation Service or the state. Accept no less under any circumstances.

Consultant's Answer:

Ask: Will our insurance cover this type of treatment? How do we find out?

Why Ask: You need to know the costs of the services recommended for your child. For example, will the costs be covered by a third party? How much will you be required to pay? Will you need to make a cash deposit? Get the answers to these questions to ensure that you select a therapist or treatment program within your budget requirements.

Consultant's Answer:

Ask: How will our family be involved in our child's treatment, including the decision for discharge and the aftercare?

Why Ask: You should expect an outpatient program to include regularly scheduled family counseling sessions. An inpatient program should provide a family component lasting a few days or weekly sessions until the end of treatment. During this time, you will participate in educational programs as well as group and family therapy.

Consultant's Answer:

Ask: How will my child continue education while in treatment?

Why Ask: If treatment is expected to last more than a week, you don't want your child to lose school time and risk the consequences. Be sure the inpatient staff includes teachers who will help keep your child current with school work.

Consultant's Answer:

Ask: How will the issue of confidentiality be handled during and after treatment?

Why Ask: Officials at the treatment facility should agree not to give out any information unless you agree and sign a release. You may also want to consider releasing information to significant others if it's in your child's best interest.

Consultant's Answer:

Ask: How long will the treatment process continue?

Why Ask: Inpatient programs usually involve a minimum of two weeks, a month, or longer depending on the severity of the problem. But this is rapidly changing. Managed care companies no longer accept this. Instead, a limited number of sessions is given and is subject to ongoing review. Also, the admission standards for treatment are more rigorous. Find out about this and weigh the information, taking into account insurance and overall budget considerations.

Consultant's Answer:

Ask: When my child is discharged from this phase of treatment, how will it be decided what types of ongoing treatment will be necessary?

Why Ask: An effective treatment program should have continuing care consisting of weekly peer group support sessions that last one to two years after inpatient treatment. The program should also include group therapy, ongoing referral to other self-help groups, and follow-up contact with clients on a regular basis, tracking their progress to ensure a successful re-entry into the community.

Consultant's Answer:

Ask: What is the program's success rate? Are statistics available that define the social, emotional, and physical growth or improvement of clients?

Why Ask: This can be a great mystery, because most inpatient programs do not conduct outcome studies of individual success rates. But ask the question anyway. You or your insurance company may be spending a good deal of money for treatment. For this kind of investment, you deserve a clear and honest response.

Consultant's Answer:

Ask: What hours does the facility operate?

Why Ask: This is not a crucial matter. But consider it, because you will want to visit your child or call about your child's well-being.

Consultant's Answer:

Ask: Is the facility's location convenient?

Why Ask: Unless you live in a remote and sparsely populated area, there's probably a treatment facility close to you. Convenience can give you better access to your child and make it financially and physically easier to participate in the treatment program.

Consultant's Answer:

Ask: Does the facility have a pleasant atmosphere in an appropriate, attractive setting?

Why Ask: Unless you can tour the facility in advance, you'll have to take the staff's word for it. Sometimes touring is difficult because of the confidential aspects of the program. Regardless, people generally respond better and work more effectively in a pleasant environment.

Consultant's Answer:

You now have enough information to make a decision about an appropriate treatment program. It's up to you to select a program that effectively meets your child's needs and your financial limitations.

Knowing What to Expect Before, During, and After Inpatient/Residential Treatment

During Inpatient/Residential Treatment

Once your child has been admitted to an inpatient program, you can usually expect treatment to last two to three weeks. Residential treatment is longer than inpatient and also more expensive. In some cases, it may be difficult to fund residential treatment through insurance alone because of the pressure and constraints of some managed care plans. Hopefully, you have learned that by now.

In treatment, your child will undergo three phases, which are described below.

- **First Phase.** If necessary, your child will be detoxified. This phase is mandatory for any child who enters the program under the influence of AOD. Moreover, if your child has recently abstained from AOD, monitoring and detoxification may be required. This process will help your child overcome the effects of AOD, safely eliminate AOD from his body, and ensure the effective adaptation of the body to normal functions without AOD. Medications and vitamins will be administered under supervision to allow minimal discomfort during the withdrawal stage. Depending on the amount and type of AOD consumed and the extent of your child's AOD abuse or dependency, the discomfort period will vary in length.
- **Second Phase.** During this stage, your child will receive a complete physical, social, and emotional assessment to determine the extent of AOD abuse or dependency and health problems. The diagnosis is conducted to correct any present health conditions and identify treatment goals and objectives. Based on the conclusions of the diagnosis, an appropriate treatment plan will be prescribed.
- **Third Phase.** The intent of the third phase is to change your child's long-term AOD abuse pattern. This process will involve individual and group therapy, educational sessions, and possible attendance of support group meetings like Alcoholics Anonymous. During this phase, your child will be educated about the nature of AOD dependency. Through this, he will identify the destructive forces in his present lifestyle and the relationship of AOD to his current problems.

Ultimately, your child will form a blueprint of expectations designed to change his long-term AOD abuse pattern into a daily routine of abstinence. He'll also determine an effective aftercare solution to ensure his successful re-entry into the community.

Throughout the treatment process, your child will experience a variety of emotions. He may feel sad, depressed, and confused in the early stages of treatment. However, as the program continues and his health and emotional stability improve, he will usually show great resilience and begin to feel more confident and act more poised. While your child is in treatment, you should educate and inform yourself about AOD dependency. With this knowledge, you will discover the strategies to effectively support and reinforce your child's aftercare program.

After Inpatient/Residential Treatment: Discharge and Aftercare Planning

The quality and success of the program depends on an effective aftercare plan that provides a blueprint for a constructive lifestyle with productive activities without the use of AOD. The aftercare plan should have detailed strategies, involving coordination and liaison with community agencies and resources, to provide the framework for your child's successful transition into the community. Most importantly, though, your child should establish meaningful relationships with people who will provide him with the emotional, psychological, and social support necessary for a sustained recovery.

The recovery phase may be a long and difficult process for your child. With an effective aftercare plan, however, the chances of your child relapsing and returning to AOD abuse can be minimized. To prevent relapse, follow-up activities must provide your child with support. These activities must also assist her in the transition and adjustment to a normal interpersonal and community life without the use of AOD. This will require a natural psychosocial support system composed of one or more of the following resources:

- participation in support group activities such as Alcoholics Anonymous or child peer group discussions focusing on recovery from drug dependency;
- individual outpatient counseling to provide emotional/psychological support, stability, and growth; and
- group and family outpatient counseling to provide social support and foster interpersonal growth for the child and her family.

Make sure that your function in the aftercare plan is clearly outlined and includes guidelines on how to monitor and evaluate your child's aftercare progress, as well as a strategy for what you should do in the event that your child relapses. You may be able to use one of the strategies in this book. This should be done only in conjunction with staff recommendations or aftercare outpatient counseling recommendations, however. Although your child's needs and choices determine which of the strategies you will use, you are in charge of the situation. Your prospects of success in preventing or stopping your child's AOD abuse are dramatically increased because the strategies have been intertwined into a proactive plan, a sensible plan of action.

Conclusion

Congratulations! You have completed this book and, as I promised, have the knowledge and a foolproof plan of action with seven strategies to prevent or stop your child's alcohol-drug abuse. You also understand how to use each strategy to accomplish this goal if your original strategy is unsuccessful. What you do, how you do it, where you go, and whom you see are based on your child's needs and choices.

Knowing that you can use the right strategy at the right time to protect your child in today's high-risk environment should ease your worries. I salute you as a loving, caring, and responsible parent/caregiver and look forward to hearing from you soon.

Appendix A
Recommended Readings

Here's a list of books that I recommend. They have been suggested and endorsed by parents like you. All of them have been used as resources for this book and appear in the bibliography. Each book has a brief description of the contents. If you use any of the books, let me know if they were helpful. And by all means, tell me about any other publication you find that would be useful to other parents.

Arterburn, S., & Burns, J. (1995). *Steering them straight.* Colorado Springs: Focus on The Family.

Helps parents recognize symptoms of potential problems such as premarital sex, suicide, and AOD abuse. Discusses several proven principles to prevent destructive teen behavior before it starts and to implement a plan of action should it occur.

Barun, K., & Basher, P. (1988). *When saying no isn't enough: How to keep the children you love off drugs.* New York: New American Library.

Provides parents with a comprehensive prevention, intervention, and treatment guide and answers questions about child and teen AOD abuse, ages 8 to 20.

Becnal, B. C. (1991). *The co-dependent parent*. San Francisco: Harper San Francisco.

The author defines the five types of co-dependent parenting: demanding, critical, overprotective, disengaging, and ineffective. Examples are offered, along with a practical course of action to deal with family denial and codependency issues.

Bloch, D. (1993). *Positive self-talk for children*. New York: Bantam Books.

Describes how to help children, from toddlers to teens, use affirmations to change negative thoughts into positive attitudes. Will help children raise their self-esteem and empower them to face life with confidence.

Bluestein, J. (1993). *Parents, teens and boundaries.* Deerfield Beach: Health Communications.

Discusses how to draw a reasonable line of expectations with testing teens. Includes techniques for avoiding conflict, resolving problems, and establishing the foundation for mutual respect.

Cline, F. (1995). *Conscienceless acts, societal mayhem, uncontrollable, unreachable youth and today's desensitized world.* Golden: Love and Logic Press.

Reveals why some children are unable to bond with others, lack a conscience, and demonstrate damaged cause-and-effect thinking. Offers parents a controversial point of view on alternatives to discipline and effectively deal with these children.

Dinkmeyer, D. C. (1997). *The parents handbook: Systematic training for effective parenting (STEP).* Circle Pines: American Guidance Service.

Contains easy-to-understand skills and practical ideas that parents can use in raising their family. A great book for the parenting library. The book is used to support and reinforce Systematic Training for Effective Parenting (STEP) workshops offered throughout the country.

Elkind, D. (1993). *Parenting your teenager in the 1990s.* Rosemost: Modern Learning Press.

Gives parents clear explanations of teen behavior and realistic suggestions about how to respond to it. Includes helpful advice on how to cope with issues such as boosting self-esteem, friendships and peer groups, depression and much more. Focuses specifically on teens and issues of the 1990s.

Freeman, J. (1989). *How to drug proof kids: A parents' guide to early prevention.* Albuquerque: The Think Shop.

A good source for useful information on drug prevention and life skills, such as feelings, self-esteem, thinking skills, assertiveness, nutrition, and decisionmaking.

Loomans, D., & Loomans, J. (1994). *Full esteem ahead: 100 ways to build self-esteem in children and adults.* Tiburon: H.J. Kramer.

Offers parents 100 practical ways to increase their children's self-esteem. Provides realistic guidelines to use the approach in a variety of ways.

Maxwell, R. (1991). *Kids, alcohol and drugs.* New York: Ballantine Books.

Discusses how to recognize potential problems and help children deal with peer, home, and school pressures. Also helps parents determine the best form of treatment if necessary.

Peele, S., & Brodsky, A. (1991). *The truth about addiction and recovery.* New York: Simon and Schuster.

Presents a controversial new approach to addiction-recovery. Identifies methods in a "Life Process Program" that the authors contend are more effective than medical treatment or 12-step programs.

Robertson, J. (1992). *Kids don't want to use drugs.* Nashville: Thomas Nelson Publishers.

Gives parents practical guidelines on how to help kids turn away from drugs. Shows parents how to recognize and meet the needs of kids to help them avoid the use of drugs.

Samenow, S. (1989). *Before it's too late: Why so many kids get into trouble.* New York: Times Books.

Parents often complain this book is always out of the library. A popular and effective book for parents with children having extensive discipline problems. Offers insight and direction in providing structure and responding to unruly kids.

Turecki, S., & Tonner, L. (1989). *The difficult child.* New York: Bantam Books.

Offers compassionate and practical advice for parents of hard-to-raise children. Shows how to manage conflict and discipline more effectively and get the support parents need.

Weston, D., & Weston, M. (1993). *Playful parenting.* Los Angeles:Tarcher/Perigee.

Offers hundreds of activities to help parents deal with the major discipline dilemmas in truly creative ways. Provides proven techniques based on the idea that children learn best through play. Addresses lying, tantrums, procrastination, and more.

Wilmes, D. J. (1988). *Parenting for prevention: How to raise a child to say no to a alcohol-drugs.* Minneapolis: Johnson Institute Publications.

Uses a positive step-by-step approach to show parents how to teach their children the life skills to resist AOD use. The theme is prevention and the approach is positive.

Youcha, G., & Sexius, J. S. (1989). *Drugs, alcohol and your children*. New York: Crown.

Describes how young people get involved with drugs. Shows parents how they can help their children get "clean." Also offers a variety of resources available for parents.

Appendix B
Resources

Organizations

Many hospitals, community colleges, and other organizations offer workshops and education classes for parents about AOD abuse and improving communication and understanding between parents and children. Contact your local library, school, or community service organization for more information.

American Council for Drug Education
164 West 74th Street
New York, NY 10017
800/488-DRUG

Provides information about drug use, develops media campaigns, reviews scientific findings, publishes books and a newsletter, and offers films and curriculum materials for pre-teens.

Families Anonymous, Inc.
P. O. Box 3475
Culver City, CA 90231-3475
800/736-9805 or 310/313-5800
Fax: 310/313-6841
http://home.earthlink.net/~famanon/index.html

Offers a 12-step, self-help program for families and friends of people with behavioral problems usually associated with drug abuse. The organization is similar in structure to Alcoholics Anonymous.

Hazelden Foundation
15245 Pleasant Valley Road
Center City, MN 55012-0176
800/257-7810 or 651/213-4000
Fax: 800/257-7800

http://www.hazelton.org/index.cfm

Distributes educational materials and self-help literature for participants in 12-step recovery programs and for the professionals who work in the field.

"Just Say No" International
1777 N. California Boulevard, Suite 210
Walnut Creek, CA 94596
800/258-2766 or 510/939-6666

Joint Commission on Accreditation of Hospitals
875 North Michigan Avenue
Chicago, IL 60611
312/642-6061

KID SAVE
800/543-7283 (24 hrs)

Referrals to shelters, mental health services, sexual abuse treatment, substance abuse, family counseling, residential care, adoption/foster care, etc.

Mothers Against Drunk Driving (MADD)
511 E. John Carpenter Freeway, Suite 700
Irving, TX 75062
800/GET-MADD or 214/744-6233
http://www.madd.org

Narcotics Anonymous (NA)
World Services Office
P.O. Box 9999
Van Nuys, CA 91409
818/773-9999
Fax: 818/700-0700
http://www.na.org

Similar to Alcoholics Anonymous, NA is a fellowship of men and women who meet to help one another with their drug dependency problems.

National Association of Alcohol and Drug Abuse Counselors (NAADAC)
1911 N. Fort Myer Drive, Suite 900

Arlington, VA 22209
800/548-0497 or 703/741-7686
Fax: 800/377-1136 or 703/741-7698
http://www.naadac.org

National Clearinghouse for Alcohol and Drug Information (NCADI)
P. O. Box 2345
Rockville, MD 20847-2345
800/SAY NOTO or 301/468-2600
Fax: 301/468-6433
http://www.health.org

NCADI is a resource for AOD information. It offers a wide variety of publications dealing with alcohol and other drug abuse.

National Council on Alcoholism and Drug Dependency
12 West 21st Street
New York, NY 10010
212/206-6770
Fax: 212/645-1690
Hope Line: 800/NCA-CALL (24-hour affiliate referral)

A national voluntary health agency that provides information about alcoholism and alcohol-related problems through more than 300 local affiliates.

National Crime Prevention Council
1700 K Street NW, 2nd Fl.
Washington, DC 20006-3817
202/466-NCPC
800/627-2911 (information requests only)

NCPC works to prevent crime and drug use in many ways, including developing materials (audiovisual, reproducible brochures, and other publications) for parents and children.

National Families in Action
Century Plaza II
2957 Clairmont Road, Suite 150
Atlanta, GA 30329
404/248-9676

Fax: 404/248-1312
http://www.emory.edu/NFIA/index.html

Publishes *Drug Abuse Update*, a quarterly journal of news and information for people interested in drug prevention; $25 for four issues.

National Federation of Parents for Drug-Free Youth, Inc.
11159-B South Towne Square
St. Louis, MO 63123
314/845-1933
http://www.healthfinder.gov/text/orgs/hr2092.htm

Sponsors the National Red Ribbon Campaign to reduce the demand for drugs and the Responsible Educated Adolescents Can Help (REACH) program to educate junior and senior high school students about drug abuse.

National Parent Teacher Association (PTA)
330 N. Wabash Avenue, Suite 2100
Chicago, IL 60611
800/307-4782
Fax: 312/670-6783
http://www.pta.org

Has "Commonsense: Strategies for Raising Alcohol- and Drug-Free Children" education program with information, resources, and easy-to-do activities for parents.

National Runaway Switchboard
3080 N. Lincoln Avenue
Chicago, IL 60657
773/880-9860
24-hour hotline: 800/621-4000
http://www.nrscrisisline.org

Offers crisis intervention, message relay between families and runaway children, referrals to community-based resources for shelter, food, health care.

Parents Resource Institute for Drug Education (PRIDE)
50 Hurt Plaza, Suite 210
Atlanta, GA 30303
800/853-7867 or 404/577-4500
http://www.prideusa.org

National S.A.F.E. Home Foundation
1333 Strad Avenue
North Tonawanda, NY 14120
800/877-1250
E-mail: safehome@buffnet
http://www.clicked.com/babytime/crib_notes/messages/25.html

Encourages parents to sign a contract stipulating that when parties are held in one another's homes, they will adhere to a strict no-alcohol-/no-drug-use rule.

Therapeutic Communities of America
1611 Connecticut Avenue NW, Suite 4-B
Washington, DC 20002
202/296-3503
Fax: 202/518-5475
http://www.echonyc.com/~sftc/tca.html

National organization of drug-free, self-help substance abuse treatment centers and rehabilitation agencies.

Toughlove
P.O. Box 1069
Doylestown, PA 18901
800/333-1069 or 215/348-7090

A national self-help group for parents, children, and communities emphasizes co-operation, personal initiative, and action; publishes a newsletter, brochures, and books; holds workshops.

Helplines

Boys Town Suicide Hotline
800/448-3000

Short-term crisis intervention and referrals to local community resources

Child Abuse National Hotline
800/252-2873 or 800/4-A-CHILD

Cocaine Hotline
800/COCAINE

Offers information, crisis intervention, and referrals for all types of drug dependency.

First Call for Help
800/468-4357

Kids' Help Phone
800/668-6868
Canadian hotline

National Adolescent Suicide Hotline
800/621-4000

National Child Abuse Hotline
800/422-4453
Multilingual crisis intervention and referrals to local social services groups

National Drug Information, Treatment, and Referral Hotline
800/662-HELP
Information and referrals to local rehabilitation centers

National Institute on Drug Abuse Helpline
800/644-6432
Science-based information on drug abuse and addiction in English and Spanish

National Suicide Hotline
888/248-2587

National Youth Crisis Hotline
800/448-4663

Nineline (sponsored by Covenant House)
800/999-9999
24-hour crisis intervention and referrals for young people under 21 and their families

Parents' Resource Institute for Drug Education Drug Information Line
404/577-4500

Bibliography

Alexander, J. (1991). *Recovery plus.* Deerfield Beach: Health Communications, Inc.

Allison, R. (1983). *Drug abuse: Why it happens and how to prevent it.* Lower Burrel: Valley Publishing.

Arterburn, S., & Burns, J. (1995). *Steering them straight.* Colorado Springs, CO: Focus on the Family.

Barun, K., & Basher, P. (1988). *When saying no isn't enough: How to keep the children you love off drugs.* New York: New American Library.

Barksdale, L.S. (1989) *Building self-esteem.* Idlewild: The Barksdale Foundation.

Bass, I. B. (1991). *The international handbook of addiction behavior.* New York: Tavistock/Routledge.

Beattie, M. (1987). *Codependent no more.* Center City, MN: Hazelden.

Beslow, A. (1989). *Change your bad habits for good.* Nashville: Abingdon Press.

Bloch, D. (1993). *Positive self-talk for children.* New York: Bantam Books.

Bluestein, J. (1993). *Parents, teens and boundaries.* Deerfield Beach: Health Communications.

Bolles, R. N. (1994). *What color is your parachute*? Berkeley, CA: Ten Speed Press.

Burns, D. (1989). *The feeling good handbook.* New York: William Morrow and Company.

Burns, D. (1993). *Ten days to self-esteem.* New York: Quill William Morrow.

Chatlos, C. (1987). *Crack: What you should know about the cocaine epidemic.* New York: Perigee Books.

Chopra, D. (1995). *Boundless energy.* New York: Harmony Books.

Christopher, J. (1989). *Unhooked.* New York: Prometheus Books.

Christopher, J. (1992). *SOS sobriety.* New York: Prometheus Books.

Cline, F. (1995). *Conscienceless acts, societal mayhem, uncontrollable, unreachable youth and today's desensitized world*. Golden, CO: Love And Logic Press.

Cudney, M., & Hardy, R. (1991). *Self-defeating behaviors*. San Francisco: Harper.

Cunningham, D., & Ramer, A. (1988). *The spiritual dimensions of healing addictions*. San Rafael, CA: Cassandra Press

Daley, D., & Miller, J. (1989). *A parent's guide to alcoholism and drug abuse*. Newport: Edgehill Publications.

Dinkmeyer, D. C. (1997). *The parents handbook: Systematic training for effective parenting (STEP)*. Circle Pines: American Guidance Service.

Duke, P. (1992). *A brilliant madness*. New York: Bantam Books.

Electronic Policy Network. (no date). Children & television: Frequently asked questions. Available on-line at http://epn.org/cme/ctatool/c_and_t.html.

Fanning, P., & O'Neil, J. T. (1996). *The addiction book*. Oakland: New Harbinger Publications, Inc.

Fleming, M., & Barry, K. (1992). *Addictive disorders*. St. Louis: Mosby-Year Book, Inc.

Freeman, J. (1989). *How to drug proof kids: A parents' guide to early prevention*. Albuquerque, NM: The Think Shop.

Freidman, H. (1991). *The self-healing personality*. New York: Henry Holt & Co.

Gabe, J. (1989). *A professional's guide to adolescent substance abuse*. Springfield, IL: Academy of Addictions Treatment.

Garner, A. (1987). *It's O.K. to say no to drugs: A parent/child manual for the protection of children*. New York: Tom Doherty Associates, 1987.

Gold, M. S. (1986). *The facts about drugs and alcohol*. New York: Bantam Books.

Gordon, T. (1970). *Parent effectiveness training (PET)*. New York: Peter H. Wyden/ Publisher.

Hart, A. (1990). *Healing life's hidden addictions*. Ann Arbor, MI: Servant Publications.

Hastings, A., Fadiman, J., & Gordon, J. (1981). *Health for the whole person*. New York: Bantam Books.

Hawkins, D. (1988). *Preparing for the drug-free years*. Seattle: Developmental Research and Programs.

Johnson, J. (1991). *It's killing our children*. Dallas: Word Publishing.

Johnson, V. (1987). *Intervention: How to help someone who doesn't want help*. Minneapolis: Johnson Institute Publications.

Jones, R. (1988). *Straight talk: Answers to questions young people ask about alcohol*. Bradenton: Human Services Institute.

King, P. (1988). *Sex, drugs, and rock and roll: Healing today's troubled youth*. Bellevue, WA: Professional Counselor Books.

Kolodny, R. C., Kolodny, N. J., Bratter, T., & Deep, C. (1984). *How to survive your adolescent's adolescence*. Boston: Little, Brown.

Krupski, A. M. (1982). *Inside the adolescent alcoholic*. Center City, MN: Hazelden.

Larson, J. (1992). *Alcoholism: The biochemical connection*. New York: Villard Books.

Lasater, L. (1988). *Recovery from compulsive behavior*. Deerfield Beach: Health Communications, Inc.

Magid, K., & McKelvey, A. (1987). *High risk children without a conscience*. New York: Bantam Books.

Maxwell, R. (1991). *Kids, alcohol and drugs*. New York: Ballantine Books.

Meyer, R. (1984). *The parent connection*. New York: Franklin Watts.

Mooney, A., Eisinberg, A., & Eisenberg, H. (1992). *The recovery book*. New York: Workman Pub. Co. Inc.

Morin, R., & Brossard, M. A. (March 4, 1997). Communication breakdown on drugs. *The Washington Post*, A1.

Nakken, C. (1988). *The addictive personality: Understanding compulsion in our lives*. New York: Harper and Row.

Nakken, C. (1988). *The addictive personality: Roots, rituals, and recovery*. Center City, MN: Hazelden Foundation.

National Parents' Resource Institute for Drug Education [PRIDE]. (1997). Results of the 1996-97 school year survey are available on-line at http://www.drugs.indiana.edu/drug_stats/pride97.html.

National Parents' Resource Institute for Drug Education [PRIDE]. (no date). Results of the 1994-95 school year survey are available on-line at http://www.mninter.net/~publish/pride.htm.

Otteson, O., Townsend, J., & Rumsey, T. (1983). *Kids and drugs: A parent's guide.* New York: CFS Publishing Corp.

Newcomb, M. B., & Bentler, P. M. (1988). *Consequences of adolescent drug use.* Newbury Park, CA: Sage Publications, Inc..

Palmer, P. (1989). *Teen esteem.* San Luis Obispo, CA: Impact Publishing.

Parents for a Drug-Free America. (no date). Results from the 1995 study are available at http://www.ndsn.org/april96/pdfa.html.

Peele, S., & Brodsky, A. (1991). *The truth about addiction and recovery.* San Luis Obispo, CA: Simon and Schuster.

Perkins, W. M., & McMurtrie-Perkins, N. (1986). *Raising drug-free kids in a drug-filled world.* Center City, MN: Hazelden.

Robertson, J. (1992). *Kids don't want to use drugs.* Nashville: Thomas Nelson Publishers.

Robinson, B. (1991). *Heal your self-esteem.* Deerfield: Health Communications.

Roy, M. (1983). *Children in the crossfire.* Deerfield Beach: Health Communications.

Ryan, E. A. (1989). *Straight talk about drugs and alcohol.* New York: Facts on File.

Samenow, S. (1989). *Before it's too late: Why so many kids get into trouble.* New York: Times Books.

Thombs, D. (1994). *Introduction to addictive behaviors.* New York: The Guilford Press.

Tobias, J. (1987). *Kids and drugs: A handbook for parents and professionals.* Annandale, MD: Panda Press.

Toffler, A. (1970). *Future shock.* New York: Random House.

Van Ost, W. C., & Van Ost, E. (1988). *Warning signs: A parent's guide to in-time intervention in drug and alcohol abuse.* New York: Warner.

Washton, A., & Boundy, D. (1989). *Willpower is not enough. Understanding and recovering from addictions of every kind.* New York: Harper and Row.

Washton, A., & Stone-Washton, N. (1991). *Step zero. Getting to recovery.* New York: HarperCollins Publishers.

Weston, D., & Weston, M. (1993). *Playful parenting.* Los Angeles:Tarcher/Perigee.

Yoder, B. (1990). *The recovery resource book.* New York: Simon and Schuster - Fireside.

Youcha, G., & Sexius, J. S. (1989). *Drugs, alcohol and your children.* New York: Crown.

About the Author

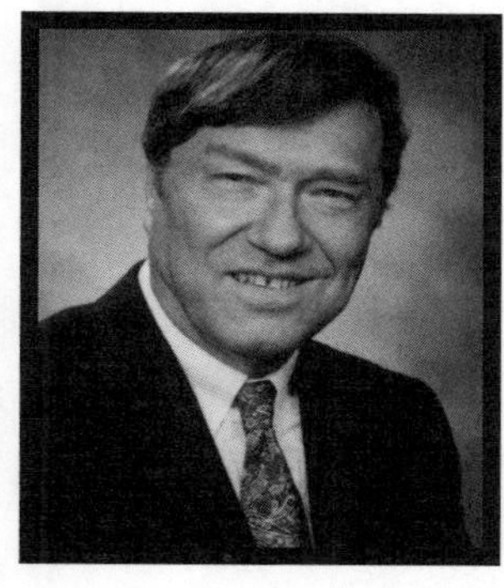

J. Stuart Rahrer, M.S. has been an author, consultant, and therapist for childhood, adolescent, and adult addiction and behavioral problems for the last 25 years. He holds a bachelor's and master's degree from Indiana University and has completed doctoral coursework in administration and counseling at the University of Arizona. Mr. Rahrer is a senior-level National Certified Addiction Counselor (NCAC II), in association with the National Association of Alcoholism and Drug Abuse Counselors, and a Certified Alcohol and Drug Addiction Counselor (CADAC-II), in the state of Indiana.

Mr. Rahrer has directed several inpatient and outpatient adolescent treatment programs and coordinated a number of alcohol-drug education and prevention projects. He has also conducted various training workshops and educational programs about child, adolescent, and adult addiction and behavioral problems for parents, child caregivers, educators, direct service providers, case managers, and professionals in mental health and corrections. His books include *The Goals for Recovery: Designing Your Own Individualized Addiction-Recovery Plan*, *Challenging How They Think: Intervention and Resolution of Adolescent Behavior Problems*, and *Stop Before Start: Early Identification and Prevention of Child Delinquent Behaviors and Conduct Problems*.

Child Welfare League of America

When Drug Addicts Have Children: Reorienting Child Welfare's Responses

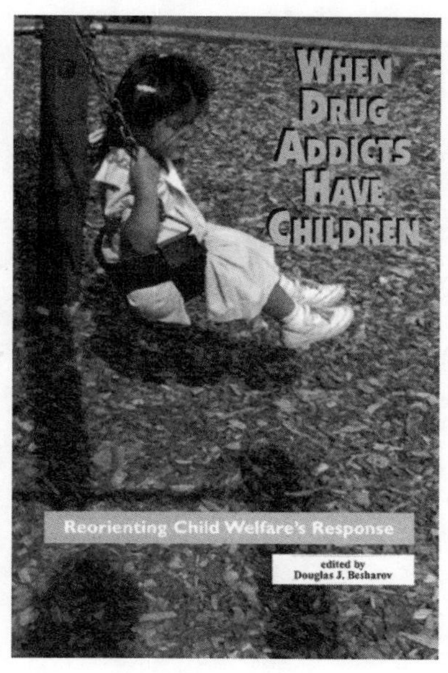

Edited by Douglas J. Besharov
with assistance from
Kristina W. Hanson
Co-published by the
American Enterprise Institute for
Public Policy Research

More than alcohol and heroin, crack cocaine threatens the well-being of hundreds of thousands of children in America today. Since 1986, it has become a fixture in the lives and neighborhoods of many low-income families.

When Drug Addicts Have Children brings together 28 program administrators, direct service providers, government officials, and scholars—all specialists in child welfare and drug abuse—in a collaborative effort to define new approaches to the complex, seemingly intractable problems associated with substance abuse and families. Readers will find a collection of provocative reports and research that calls for a redical new approach to the care and treatment of children abused and neglected by their drug-addicted parents. A *must* for all addiction and child welfare professionals!

To Order: 1994/0-87868-561-8 Stock #5618 $15.95

Write:	CWLA P.O. Box 2019 Annapolis Junction, MD 20701	Call:	800/407-6273 301/617-7825
E-mail:	cwla@pmds.com	Fax:	301/206-9789

Please specify stock #5618. Bulk discount policy (not for resale): 10-49 copies 10%, 50-99 copies 20%, 100 or more copies 40%. Canadian and foreign orders must be prepaid in U.S. funds. MasterCard/Visa accepted.